Dr. Johnson provides a way for parents to help their children cope with today's culture of sex and raise them to have a healthy sexual awareness that is appropriate to their age. A realistic, experience-based approach for parents concerned about the impact of today's culture of sex on their children.

> —Kenneth Prescott, MSW, LCSW, Chair, Los Angeles Sex Offender Roundtable Secretary, California Coalition of Sexual Offending

Toni's book is a necessary resource for anyone who works with children who have sexual behavior problems. It provides a very good description of how to identify behaviors that are normal and those that are of concern, and of how to identify the seriousness of those behaviors that are of concern. I am going to require all of my staff members to read it!

> —Barry Jenkins, ACSW, Peyton Anderson Center Director, The Methodist Home for Children and Youth, Macon, Georgia

Dr. Johnson offers a balanced view of childhood sexual behavior that reflects psychological conflict along with an explanation of normal childhood sexual behavior. Her book provides expert examples and tools to help us respond to the spectrum of these behaviors.

> —Michael Durfee, M.D., Psychiatrist, Los Angeles, California, International expert on child abuse and preschool sexual abuse

Where I failed as a father and child psychiatrist and sexologist in really listening to the sexuality of my daughter, I succeeded with the help of Dr. Johnson's thrilling new book as a grandfather to my grandson.

> —Frits Bruisma, M.D., Child Psychiatrist and Sexologist, the Netherlands

Give your child something wonderful, read this book! It offers clear practical advice on how to use everyday situations to talk naturally about sex with children. Excellent.

> —Dr. Paul W. Miller, MB, BCh, BAO, DMH, MRCPsych., National Health Service Psychiatrist, Northern Ireland

This is a much-needed book that puts into perspective the range of childhood sexual behaviors. Parents will find it straightforward and full of helpful specifics about encouraging healthy sexuality. Professionals will find it an asset in helping parents cope with the process of childhood sexual exploration.

> —Barbara Jones Smith, Ph.D., Licensed Clinical
> Psychologist and Board Certified Sex
> Therapist, Traverse City, Michigan

Dr. Johnson's book is an important collection of our knowledge and evidence in the area of childhood sexuality. She describes in detail the wide scope of children's normal sexual behaviors from birth to age 12. Her descriptions of assessing and addressing behaviors, and, if need be, changing them, are simple, clear, and down-to-earth.

> —Carolle Trembley, Registered Psychologist,
> Founding Member of Child and Adolescent
> Perpetrators Treatment System in Canada

A helpful and practical text by a well-respected and experienced clinical psychologist. I find this book informative, systematic in approach, and highly accessible.

> —Helen Chan, Ph.D., Clinical Psychologist and
> mother, Hong Kong

Separating normal sexual behaviors of children from those which are outside the normal, is always difficult. For those like myself who are frequently unsure when faced with such behaviors, Dr. Johnson gives clear, factual and simple descriptions of these problems and their causes.

> —Robin Fancourt, M.D., Pediatrician, New
> Plymouth, New Zealand

Dr. Johnson's work is impressive and manages to combine an appreciation of the complexity of sexuality and children's sexual behaviors with a brevity and clarity of presentation that makes issues accessible. This book takes readers through a process of calm examination and explanation toward a point where helpful, informed interventions with children become possible.

> —Jim Ennis, Child Protection Studies,
> Department of Social Work, University of
> Dundee, Scotland

Understanding Your Child's Sexual Behavior

WHAT'S
NATURAL
AND
HEALTHY

Toni Cavanagh Johnson, Ph.D.

NEW HARBINGER PUBLICATIONS, INC.

Distributed in the U.S.A. by Publishers Group West; in Canada by Raincoast Books; in Great Britain by Airlift Book Company, Ltd.; in South Africa by Real Books, Ltd.; in Australia by Boobook; and in New Zealand by Tandem Press.

Copyright © 1999 by Toni Cavanagh Johnson, Ph.D.
New Harbinger Publications, Inc.
5674 Shattuck Avenue
Oakland, CA 94609

Cover design by Poulson/Gluck Design
Text design by Michele Waters

Library of Congress Catalog Card Number: 98-68756
ISBN 1-57224-141-1 Paperback

New Harbinger Publications' Website address: www.newharbinger.com

01   00   99

10   9   8   7   6   5   4   3   2   1

First printing

This book is dedicated to my husband, Bill, and my three grown children, Matthew, Taj, and Alexis

Contents

Acknowledgments

Over the years many professionals have contributed to my thinking about children and their sexual behaviors and this knowledge is reflected in this book. They are far too numerous to list here and they have been mentioned in other books that I have written. I value all of their help and knowledge.

I want to acknowledge all of the children and their families with whom I have worked. They are a source of inspiration and knowledge. I hope they have learned as much from me as I have from them.

I want to thank the following people who gave me feedback on what I wrote while I was in the process of writing and rewriting. Various members of the Association for the Treatment of Sexual Abusers read different chapters and offered me their feedback. They were marvelous for their knowledge and quick responses. Many people even endured reading several rewrites of chapters. Writing a book can be a very lonely adventure. Doing this book with the feedback made it an exciting process. Ron Kokish, Kerry Lindorfer, Susan Rich, and Carolle Trembley read virtually everything and gave me a tremendous amount of feedback. Other ATSA members who helped greatly are Bill Ballantyne, Mary E. S. Bennett, Janis Bremer, Frits Bruisma, Ed Dawson, Carol A. Deel, Niki Delson, Robert E. Freeman-Longo, Eliana Gil, Fran Henry, Barbara Jones Smith, Paul Rock Krech, Jessica Lay, Paul D. Lowder, Paul W. Miller, Jacqueline Pei, Gail Ryan, and Theo Seghorn.

I needed a balance of people to help me. Many friends and relatives provided feedback from a nonclinical or research orientation. These people know children. I am very grateful to them for their time and energy. Many thanks go to Lucinda Denton, Susan Denton, Taj Johson, Alexis Johnson, Patricia Cavanagh McKee, Judy Cavanagh Stoll, Ann Fink, Julie Stevens, Marlene Stevens, Elizabeth Warner, and Rella Warner.

There are many members of the California Professional Society on the Abuse of Children (CAPSAC) who are always willing to help me. I am especially grateful to Colleen Friend, Mike Hertica, and Michelle Winterstein.

I also had the help of a man who sexually offended against children for many years. We have been in contact for several years since I did seven hours of videotaped interviews with him and his therapist. The interviews served as the basis for teaching others about sexual offenders. Jim Hosch was caught for molesting children and spent several years in prison where he received good sex offender specific therapy. He is working to help others understand sexual offenders. He was a great help to me in the last chapter of the book. Jim gave me many ideas that I incorporated into the text. He wants parents to know how to spot sexual offenders and children to know how to not be trapped by them. I am grateful to him for using his knowledge to benefit (instead of exploit) children at this time in his life.

Introduction

When your child is engaging in sexual behaviors, it can be difficult to decide when the sexual behavior is natural and healthy and when it may be an indication of some distress or disturbance.

This book is for the parents, grandparents, teachers, day care workers, and others who are curious about children's sexual behaviors. If you are a psychologist, clinical social worker, school psychologist, school counselor, nurse, pediatrician, family care physician, child protective services worker, social worker in a foster family agency, or someone who works with children in any capacity, you will also find that this book can teach you to distinguish *natural* and *healthy childhood* sexuality from *disturbed* sexuality.

How Can This Book Help Me?

Information is provided throughout this book helping you to recognize and modify problematic sexual behavior. You will learn specific ways to foster a healthy sexual development for your children. Also included are guidelines for you and your children on how to effectively communicate with one another regarding sex. And finally, there are helpful strategies for reducing the risk of child sexual abuse.

Does the Age of My Child Matter?

The ages of the children discussed in this book are from birth to approximately twelve years old, or the age at which a particular child moves into pubertal sexuality. This will be different for each child. This book deals with prepubertal sexuality, which is fundamentally different from postpubertal sexual development. After the sex-related hormones come into play during puberty, there are substantial changes in the body and concomitant changes in the feelings and thoughts of children. The orientation of young children regarding sex is curiosity about their bodies and the differences between their bodies and others.

Young children often become fascinated by gender differences and the social relationships between males and females. Pubertal children and adolescents feel sexual and look for ways to explore genital pleasure and touching for erotic gratification. Dating and sexual contact become priorities for adolescents—in fact, sexual desire may dominate their thinking. The priorities for prepubertal childhood sexuality, on the other hand, are far less genital, less erotic, and more exploratory.

Child Sexuality Versus Adult Sexuality

Language becomes a problem when writing about behaviors of young children related to sex and sexuality. What terminology is accurate? If I use the term *childhood sexual behaviors*, am I distinguishing between adult and child sexual behavior? Yes, because "childhood" is in front of sexual. But will you, the reader, remember to distinguish between adult and child sexuality? Perhaps you won't. Is this a problem? Yes, because many adults confuse adult and child sexuality and therefore interpret it incorrectly.

Is there another term that would continuously remind you of this difference? One possibility is the term *presexual*. However, this term isn't in current use and is not truly accurate. Children are sexual but not in the genitally-focused way of adults where arousal and pleasure are the goals.

The term *sensual* better describes the types of feelings experienced by children. Children feel pleasurable sensations from genital touch as with other types of touch, such as rubbing their ears, mouth, back, legs, twirling hair between their fingers, sucking thumbs, toes, and lollipops. But not all of the behaviors of children that are related to sex and sexuality can be classified as sensual behaviors because so many of the behaviors have to do with *discovering gender differences* and *studying sex roles*. Alas, the term childhood sexual behaviors will be used. Therefore, remember to distinguish between adult and child sexuality.

The reason this difference between adult and child sexuality is important to stress is because parents tend to confuse their own thoughts and feelings about sex and sexuality with those of their children. If they see their child masturbating they may equate this with their own behavior and be concerned about the child's fantasies. A foster parent seeing his or her seven-year-old foster child "humping" another child may think that child is trying to get sexual satisfaction.

Very few young children seek sexual arousal and pleasure. Sexual arousal and pleasure akin to adult sexual experiences are uncommon among young children and are more likely to occur the closer the child gets to puberty. It's far safer for parents to assume that the child is experimenting with behaviors and gender roles rather than seeking adult-like sexual relationships and sexual stimulation. If a parent isn't sure, he or she should listen carefully to what his or her child says rather than assume he or she know.

It's also a good idea for parents to think back to their own sexual experiences when prepubertal, and differentiate between childhood, adolescent, and adult experiences. Parents should also remember that their child is a unique individual and is not a clone of either parent. Listen to your child and value his or her individuality.

How Will I Know What Is "Normal"?

There are three areas I will cover related to the sexual behaviors of children. The first is *natural* and *healthy sexual behaviors*. I will define this type of behavior and give lots of examples. In addition, you'll find charts that describe natural and healthy behaviors in the first column and then show that behavior in the next two columns being a behavior of increasing concern.

For instance, some preschool children play doctor, inspecting each other's bodies. This is within the realm of natural and healthy sexual curiosity. Yet, if the preschool child plays doctor frequently after repeatedly being told "no," there is a reason for concern. In natural and healthy sexual play, when children are told to stop they either stop or continue but hide the behavior. The third column in the chart indicates that there is another level of increased concern if the child forces another child to play doctor or to take off their clothes.

I will talk about characteristics of children's sexual behaviors that should raise the parents' concern and give lots of examples. In some cases I recommend seeking professional assistance. I encourage you to talk to your children about sexual issues and give you guidelines on how to do this. I have also included hints for your children or how to talk to you.

When you finish the book you should have a far greater understanding of children's sexual behaviors and have sound ideas about what to do. Many parents worry that their child may have been sexually abused if they are engaging in worrisome sexual behaviors. I will discuss this as well as give you lots of ideas on how to reduce your child's risk of being sexually abused.

CHAPTER 1

What Are Natural and Healthy Sexual Behaviors During Childhood?

As life grows more complex, we're all trying to assure the safety of our children. Since the early 1980s we have been bombarded with information about child sexual abuse. We worry that our child may be abused. Some parents who witness their child being sexual with another child worry that this is abnormal and is the result of being sexually abused.

Other parents may not ascribe sexual abuse as the cause, but may be upset that their child is being sexual and feel that this is bad behavior. All parents struggle with what is normal, or "natural and healthy." This chapter will provide examples of natural and healthy sexual behavior. I start with my definition of natural and healthy sexual behavior in prepubertal children. Chapter 2 will take this definition and explain it in more detail.

Natural and healthy sexual exploration during childhood is an *information-gathering process* wherein children explore each other's and their own bodies by *looking and touching* (for example, looking in the mirror or playing doctor), as well as *explore gender roles and behaviors* (for example, playing house). Children involved in natural and healthy sexual play are of *similar age, size,* and *developmental status* and participate on a *voluntary basis*. While siblings often engage in mutual sexual exploration, most sex play is between children who have an ongoing *mutually enjoyable* play and/or school *friendship*. The sexual behaviors are limited in type and frequency and occur in several periods of a child's life.

A child's interest in sex and sexuality is balanced by curiosity about other aspects of his or her life. And while natural and expected sexual exploration may result in embarrassment, children are not usually left feeling anger, shame, fear, or anxiety. In most cases, if children are discovered in sexual exploration and instructed to stop, the behavior ceases, at least in the view of adults. The healthy feelings of children regarding their sexual behavior is usually *lighthearted, spontaneous, silly* and *giggly*.

Many children experience pleasurable sensations from genital touching. Some children experience sexual arousal, and some children experience orgasms. While sexual arousal and orgasms are possible at any age, they are more likely to occur in older children entering puberty than in younger children.

So What Are Children Doing?

Now you've been introduced to the main concepts that define healthy childhood sexual behavior. The definition of natural and healthy sexual exploration in children provides you with a foundation for understanding children's sexual development. However, each of these areas will be explained in more in detail in chapter 2.

Following are some common stories of children and their sexual exploration. As you read these scenarios, ask yourself if they fit your definition of healthy, sexual behaviors.

The Closet Kissers in First Grade

Pablo and Sally, two six-year-olds who are classmates and play handball together, were alone in the large closet where first-graders hang up their jackets. "Wanna try it?" Pablo said to Sally. What an idiot, Sally thought. What is he talking about? Try what? Looking puzzled, she said curtly, "What are you talking about?" Pablo winked at her. She looked at him like he was crazy. Pablo winked again thinking she doesn't get it yet. Sally walked out of the closet thinking, "Boys, they're all weird."

Pablo had seen his teenage brother with his girlfriend Joan in the backyard the night before. Pablo wasn't exactly sure what happened, but he thought that his brother said something to Joan, winked at her, and then she kissed him. Undaunted by Sally's rebuff, Pablo determined to spy on his brother and Joan again. He really wanted to kiss a girl.

Penis Delight for a Second-Grader

Mark was showering with his seven-year-old son Kevin, when Kevin asked why his penis was so big. Mark told Kevin that his was small when he was seven and that penises get bigger as the body grows. Satisfied, Kevin said he would wait but would really like a bigger one now.

The next day Kevin was in the bathroom while his mother was showering. He looked behind the shower curtain and raised his voice to ask his mother a question. His mother asked him to give her privacy and explained that she would talk to him when she finished her shower and dressed. Kevin persisted in looking and finally left when his mother raised her voice a bit.

When she was dressed, Kevin's mother talked to him. Kevin wanted to know if she had a penis. She said, "No, girls don't have penises." Kevin looked very worried and asked, "Did you lose it?" Finding this amusing, Kevin's mother smiled and said, "No, I didn't lose it. Girls don't have penises." Kevin, concerned, said, "What a shame, penises are so much fun. I'll try to get you one."

Love Notes in Third Grade

The teacher in a third grade classroom caught a girl sending a boy a note. It said, "I want to have a sex with you." The teacher asked the little girl to explain the note. The little girl said, "I'm not sure what it means, but I heard my sister talking on the phone to her boyfriend last night about sex and it sounded like fun."

The Trash Mouths in Fourth Grade

Michelle taught a fourth grade class. One morning she entered the room and found mostly quiet children, but also some snickering ones. Looking around she saw that "bon" was prominently written on the board. Michelle asked for someone to read the syllable. By this time most of the children were giggling and some were looking uncomfortable. No one volunteered to read.

Michelle said, "Bon, I wonder what that word means." Laughter escaped from some of the children. Addressing the children who were laughing, she said with a smile, "Was it bon you meant to write, or bone?" Snickers and giggles and coughing and embarassment followed. None of the children offered an answer.

Michelle handled her students' sexual experimentation by giving them a lesson in spelling. "When you're trying to get the long 'o' sound, you have to put an 'e' at the end of the word. So, with the syllable 'bon,' if you wanted it to be 'bone' you would put an 'e.' Is that what you wanted to spell?" No one answered. "Who can tell me what 'bone' means?" Then there were gales of laughter from some of the more savvy students. Michelle directed her comments to them and explained, "Bone is a slang way to refer to a part of the body. If you're going to use slang, I suggest you learn how to spell so people don't make fun of you. If you use the proper words, you can be sure that people will know what you are talking about. Penis is spelled p-e-n-i-s. Are there any questions?" There was not a sound in the room!

Flying Objects in Fifth Grade

Several boys and girls were flying little "bombs" and paper airplanes to one another in Max's fifth grade class one morning. The children became so involved in their play that no one noticed when their teacher, Max, moved to the back of the room quickly and captured four of the missiles. The children looked panicked. Max asked for more of the flying objects. He was given two more and one child seemed to be swallowing something! He asked all of these children to stay in the class during recess so that they could "talk."

The next twenty-five minutes were torturous for the children. They were afraid to even try to communicate with one another. The other children in the class were equally sedate knowing that their friends were caught.

After all of the other children had gone to recess, Max brought out the "bombs" and paper airplanes and asked, "What were these for?" One of the children, Dan, said, "Oh, we were being rude. We're sorry. We won't do it again. If you want, I'll throw those away for you." Max thanked Dan but said that instead perhaps he should open one of the "bombs" for Max to read. Dan said that he didn't think the bombs really needed to be opened. Max indicated he would open them. Dan reluctantly agreed. "Okay, I'll do it." He opened the first "bomb" and read out loud, "I love you."

Max asked to see the paper. The paper actually read, "I want to f--- you." Max told Dan that he wasn't looking for a translation, especially an incorrect one. The other messages read, "You're really hung," "Did you see those tits on Mrs. Walsh?", "Sex feels good," and "Mrs. Smith [the principal] must be on the rag."

Max spent the rest of recess talking to his students about the meaning being transmitted in each message. He explained that it is best to see people as a whole and not as "sexual parts." He also talked about respecting others. Max kept the discussion lighthearted and frank. The children were relieved and understood what he was saying.

However, some of the children's parents were less understanding than the teacher. They punished their children; two were given harsh spankings. When children engage in "misbehavior," parents often want to decide what their children need to learn. Max targeted that well. Some of the parents shut down further communication about sexual topics with their children because of their own disproportionate anger over the incident and lack of understanding of children's natural and healthy interest in sexuality as they move into adolescence.

The Sixth-Grader's Slumber Party

Ten eleven-year-old girls celebrated Trina's birthday with a sleepover in Trina's converted basement. They laughed and giggled, played love songs, and talked about boys. They used every bad word they'd ever heard and pretended to be movie stars. By 3 A.M. most of the girls were sound asleep. But two of the girls, Lisa and Moira, stayed up talking about boys, sex, and contraception. They were trying to figure out from all the bits of information that they had what contraceptive they would use when they got older and had sex. That is, if they decided to have sex. Neither was truly convinced they wanted to have sex because boys were so "gross."

As they talked they asked each other about female genitalia. Moira wanted to know if Lisa had ever explored her "pussy"? What was the other's vagina like? Moira, giggling hysterically, told Lisa that people called the flaps on the outside of the vagina "lips." "Nobody is ever going to kiss my 'lips'," she said, buckling over with laughter. Other girls began to complain about the noise they were making and so they went in the bathroom. While in the bathroom Moira asked Lisa to go in the shower while she used the toilet because she wanted privacy. Lisa gladly went in the shower and looked the other way. As Moira was urinating, Lisa laughed and asked if Moira had ever wished she had a penis so she could spray like the boys. This sent them both into uncontrollable laughter.

After they regained some composure Moira asked if Lisa had ever tried to see inside herself using a mirror. Lisa said she tried but couldn't really see. Moira then said,"Want to look inside me and then I will look inside you?" "Gross," said Lisa, and then almost immediately said, "Let's." "Do you promise never to tell anyone?" They both agree that they would never tell anyone. They explored each other's vaginal area with all of the seriousness of medical doctors.

What Do You Think?

Some parents reading these stories will be unsure that these children's behaviors are within the natural and healthy range. Some parents will laugh and remember doing similar things. Other parents will have mixed reactions. Remember that you have developed your own standards of acceptable behaviors based on personal experiences.

The purpose of the stories is to illustrate common sexual behaviors of children in this era. The stories aren't to tell you what you should accept for your children but to demonstrate what is within the natural and healthy range of expectable behaviors for young children. You need to teach your children what is acceptable according to your beliefs. Just be sure of why you believe the way you do and be able to explain it to your child.

About the Research in This Book

Studying children's sexual behavior is difficult because most occurs in secret. Few children tell adults what they do. And when children are discovered, if they receive a negative reaction, they generally try to keep the details to themselves. Even if they don't receive a negative reaction, just the questioning can make them feel uncomfortable.

To overcome the paucity of direct observation and detailed descriptions, I use several of my recent surveys throughout the book to supplement the description of natural and healthy sexual behavior in children. You will find the results of two particular studies in the boxed sections within the chapters. One study is of approximately four hundred college students across the United States. The other is of approximately four hundred mental health professionals and child welfare workers also across the United States. The participants in both of these studies were asked about their sexual behaviors when they were twelve years old and younger. For a detailed account of the studies, refer to the appendix at the back of this book.

CHAPTER 2

Understanding Children's Sexual Exploration and Curiosity

This chapter will explain natural and healthy childhood sexual behaviors in detail providing statistical data gathered from adults remembering back to their childhood sexual experiences. Chapter 3 will help you understand the characteristics of problematic sexual behavior during childhood.

Some Common Exploration Practices

Remember, children's natural and healthy sexual exploration is an *information gathering process*. It involves children exploring and touching their own bodies. When trying to understand their body and sexuality, children naturally use their own bodies as a map. Just as they stick their fingers in their ears, noses, and mouths, children explore what you may call the "private parts" of their bodies.

When you're changing the diapers of your children or bathing them, for instance, you may see your child touch his penis or put her finger on her labia. This is a good opportunity for you to name this part of the body. "That is your penis. That is a private part of your body." "Those are called the labia. That is a private part of your body." It is good for you to take every available opportunity to teach about the body parts and help the children develop an accurate vocabulary. This encourages open discussion about sexual topics.

You may find your child peeking when you're in the bathroom or trying to listen outside your bedroom. This can provide the opportunity to ask if he or she has any questions and indicate your willingness to answer them while also teaching them about privacy: "I will gladly answer any questions you have but everyone deserves not to be spied on." If your child starts to fondle his or her genitals when you're present you can say, "That is for when you are alone."

Forty-eight percent of the college students surveyed said they looked at their body in the mirror when they were between the ages of eleven and twelve, and 23% did this when they were between six and ten. Thirty-seven percent of the students said they became more detailed in their exploration and explored their bodies, including their genitals, when they were between eleven and twelve years old. Thirty-one percent said they did this when they were between the ages of six and ten. Twenty-six of the eleven- and twelve-year-olds and 16% of the six- to ten-year-olds said they had fondled their genitals.

Looking and Touching Others

As part of their information gathering, children explore each other's bodies by *looking* and *touching*. These are the standard ways in which children gather information about each other's bodies. By looking and touching they begin to build an understanding of what the body looks like, what differences exist between boys and girls, and what it feels like to touch another's body. It's not uncommon for children to be caught in the bathroom or in a bedroom or playroom at home examining each other's bodies. Although this often causes teachers and parents dismay, this is a time-honored learning method. Children like to see and touch sand, jello, mud, caterpillars, sparkly items, penises, and vaginas. Each of these spark an interest in children. The most curious children often do the most exploring—curiosity is at the heart of learning.

In the study of college students, 17% said that they "touched or explored the private parts of another child" when they were twelve and younger. In the survey of 352 mental health and child welfare workers, 30% said they showed their "private parts" to another child, and 46% said that they "played doctor."

Exploring Through the Media

As part of their information gathering, children look at *magazines, videos, books,* explore the *Internet,* and *peek at others.* Such an abundance of material with sexual content has probably never been more available to children. Network television and cable television with music videos, talk shows about sex, and call-in sex shows are an enormous source of information and misinformation. Radio has call-in talk shows whose primary topics are sex. Children with radios and ear phones can listen in the wee hours of the night without detection.

You probably want to try to monitor your children's intake of information from the various media. This is frequently impossible. Therefore, it's helpful for you to have frequent and frank discussions about sexual topics to monitor what your children know. Many parents watch a few shows a week with their children and use what is on the television to stimulate discussion. A lot of shows targeted to children show dating and kissing and other sexual topics. You can use the TV to reinforce values you accept or to point out ones you don't, or ask your child what he or she thinks about what is being portrayed. Television and other media are natural vehicles for talking about sexual topics with children. You can search for "teachable moments."

Be aware of what you watch when your children are around. Not only does this give children permission to watch but it also models what is of interest and what is acceptable to their parents. Children learn from their parents. If you're watching a show or video portraying something you don't approve of, you can use the opportunity to teach your child. "Men should not be mean to women like that. I hope she leaves him. Women should not put up with that kind of abuse." "It looks as if that teenager is getting in a lot of trouble. I wonder if his parents need to help him more. Kids should tell their parents when they have problems. I hope you will tell me or Mommy if you have any worries. We're always here to help. Sometimes kids are afraid to tell if they do something wrong but it's better to tell and get our help. That's what we're here for."

When college students were asked about their primary sources of sex education, 68% said friends, 55% parents, 54% sex education in school, 39% said books, 34% television. Thirteen percent said sex education came from pornographic material. Forty-four percent of the eleven- to twelve-year-olds said they looked at "dirty pictures," 25% of the six to ten-year-olds did this.

What's All the Fuss About?

In natural and healthy sexual play or exploration children are generally excited and feel silly and giggly. It is fun and enticing. Early on children seem to understand that sexual exploration should be done secretively. It's important for you to try not to make your children feel badly if you catch them exploring. A calm tone of voice and short statements are best. (This is explained more in chapter 10.)

Unfortunately, some parents make their children feel ashamed about their desire for sexual knowledge and touching. This can cast a negative shadow over their sexual development that may deter them from further exploration. Learning about sex and feeling confident and happy about it is part of healthy sexual development.

Prior to the 1980s when we knew less about the sexual abuse of children, there may have been a more relaxed attitude amongst many parents about their children's sexual behaviors. We now live in a time when many parents worry that if their child is engaging in sexual behaviors the child has been sexually abused.

There is a tension in our society that may infect the sexual play of children. This can be a great loss to children for their sexual development and for their attitude toward sex and sexuality. Sexual curiosity and play should be lighthearted. Children can have a great deal of fun exploring what it means to be a man or woman. If children are looking at each other's bodies and their behavior doesn't fit the problematic characteristics listed in chapter 3, you'll be better off not making a big deal about it.

I am concerned that some children have begun to equate touching private parts with abuse. While this is abuse under certain circumstances, it is not under *all* circumstances. For instance, during childhood many children play doctor or touch another child's private parts: Do we want children to think this is abusive?

In the mid- and late 1980s when it was discovered that children molested other children, there was a surge of *mislabeling sexual exploration* as *sexual molestation*. This concern on the part of adults can find its way to children and diminish their positive feelings about sexual exploration.

When children grow into adolescence they'll likely engage in some genital touching: How will they know that isn't abuse? Some children may even construe sexual contact between adults as abuse.

You can help by listening carefully to any comments or questions your children may have about sex and sexuality to make sure that they're not getting a negative message about sex.

Another concern is that sexual touch is often equated with "bad touch." Some prevention programs leave children with this message. As a result, children may misconstrue their natural curiosity to touch and explore as "bad."

When they were engaging in sexual behaviors alone, 40% of the college students said they felt good or fine, 34% felt silly or giggly. When they were engaging with other children in sexual behaviors, 37% felt good or fine, 48% felt silly or giggly. It seems that it is more fun to engage in sexual behaviors with other children. When asked if they felt "excited (not sexually)," 21% said "yes" when they engaged in sexual behaviors alone and 24% said "yes" for mutual behaviors with one other child.

College students also indicated less positive feelings. When participating in sexual behaviors alone, 32% felt confused, 30% felt guilty, 16% felt scared, 13% felt bad. When involved in mutual sexual behaviors with one other child, 27% felt confused, 21% felt guilty, 21% felt scared, and 8% felt bad. These data indicate that behaving sexually creates a lot of feelings in children and many are not positive. Feelings of confusion and guilt are quite high in children who engage in sexual behaviors. Parents do not want to increase these feelings for natural and healthy sexual exploration.

For example, a colleague who is a psychologist in Michigan described the following scene she witnessed in a preschool. As she was observing the four-year-olds on their playground, she saw three children playing together. They were giggling and having a good time. After a few minutes the little boy kissed each of the girls on the cheek. One of the little girls turned around and shouted "sex abuse" toward where her teacher was standing.

You can be a good model for your children by showing affection in front of them, such as lighthearted kissing and hugging.

Bathroom Humor and Games

Another aspect of typical childhood curiosity is a delight in *bathroom humor* and *games*, an interest that sometimes flusters adults. Three ten-year-old boys, for example, threw the staff at one elementary school into conflict when they were discovered playing in the bathroom. One of the children was "creating designs in the toilet bowl with his urine," while his two friends were seeing which boy could stand the farthest away while directing urine from his penis into the bowl. The principal was convinced the behavior was "perverted" and suggested that the children be removed from school (Morgan 1984 #80).

Despite the principal's alarm, this is an excellent example of healthy—if, perhaps, mischievous—childhood behavior. The typical affect of children regarding normal behaviors related to sexuality is lighthearted and spontaneous. These boys were trying out something fun. They were exploring the capabilities of their bodies.

Sex Is Just a Part of the Whole Picture

The sexual behavior of children engaged in the normal process of childhood exploration is balanced with *curiosity about other parts of their universe*. They want to know how babies are made as well as why the sun disappears. They want to explore the physical differences between males and females as well as figure out how to get their homework done quickly so they can play outside. Children often go through periods when they seem to be always interested in sexual things, and then it becomes less prominent. Some children's sexual interest never becomes known to parents and some young children do not become interested.

Which Children Explore?

There are *wide differences* in the *sexual development* and interest of children. Some theorists, including Freud, have thought that all children engage in sexual behaviors but this is not the case. In fact, there may be a substantial number of children who don't show any particular interest in sexual topics during childhood.

Fifty-seven percent of the college students said they had engaged in solitary sexual behaviors when they were twelve years and younger and 60% said they engaged in sexual behaviors with one other child during this period of childhood. Twenty percent said they engaged in sexual behaviors with two or more children. Therefore, it's obvious that not all children take part in sexual behaviors during their childhood.

The college student data also indicates a wide variation in the number of times they engaged in any of the behaviors. While most of the students only participated in the behaviors one to eight times, four students in the sample indicated engaging in behaviors hundreds of times.

Likewise, children show different levels of interest. If your child is very interested in sexual topics and sexual touch, this may simply be a reflection of his or her inborn drives. If your child has no interest in sexual topics or exploration, this may also be a reflection of inborn characteristics.

Thirteen percent of the college students said they remembered dreaming about sex when they were between eleven and twelve, only 3% remembered this when they were between six and ten years old.

Friends

Sexual behaviors occur mainly between children who have an *ongoing mutual play* or *friend* relationship. Childhood friends explore caves, woodlands, video games, how to light matches, make cookies, play football, and play sexually together. This type of exploration does happen between brothers and sisters who are close in age or who don't live near their friends, but it's more likely to occur between friends.

This is the same with sexual contact. There is noncoercive sexual contact between siblings that is still natural and healthy but most children pick someone outside their family with whom they have an ongoing play relationship. Since behaving sexually is taboo to most parents, your children probably want to make sure they aren't going to be told on. This is why they're more likely to sexually experiment with their friend than with a sibling who may get angry with a sibling and tell "Mommy."

Overwhelmingly, when young children engage in mutual sexual behaviors, they choose friends rather than relatives or siblings. The choice of friends is six times more likely than siblings or relatives. It's extremely rare, however, that a child would engage in sexual behavior with someone they didn't know.

Who Are Your Child's Friends?

Children involved in natural and healthy exploration are generally of *similar age, size,* and *developmental level*. The average age difference is about six months between children who are experimenting sexually. For instance, if your child is eight years old he or she will probably engage in sexual behaviors with someone who is between seven-and-a-half and eight-and-a-half years old.

Perhaps your child is large or small for his or her age. In this case, however, size isn't relevant. Likewise, if your child is ten but has an emotional age of six and plays with six-year-olds, this might also be an exception to the age and size difference as most sexual behavior between young children occurs between friends. If your child lives in an area without peer-age friends, he or she may engage in sexual behaviors with nonpeer age friends.

Checking Out the Gender Roles

Gender roles is an area of high exploration. Children are very interested in male and female roles. The stereotypical male and female roles are beginning to erode but boys playing bad guys, and girls playing with dolls, is still seen in preschools throughout the United States. Trying on gender roles can also move into playing house, with one person playing mommy and the other daddy. This can turn into divorce or the exploration of the roles of mommies and daddies in "baby-making."

Twelve percent of the mental health and child welfare professionals said they engaged in "humping" or simulating intercourse. Eighteen percent of the college students also said they partook in this behavior.

Exploring other gender roles and clothes has become culturally more acceptable for little girls but remains controversial for boys. Boys trying on girls' clothes and exploring their sex role behaviors are not highly uncommon up until the age of about five or six. Once children enter school, boys tend to consolidate their sex role characteristics although they aren't as rigid as they used to be. Boys interested in dance, cooking, poetry, sewing, and other traditionally female-oriented interests are no longer the subject of intense negative appraisal.

If you are worried that your child's sex role development is different than other children his or her age, you may want to consult your pediatrician or a licensed mental health practitioner with advanced study in child development. Never try to make your children ashamed of who they are or how they behave, and always remember that respect for your child is the most important thing.

If your child is being ridiculed by his or her peers, he or she needs your support. Some children also need to become more aware of their behavior and make choices. Ridicule doesn't generally bring behavioral change (for any behavior) over the long run, yet it manages to destroy self-esteem and the relationship between the person doing the ridiculing and the person ridiculed.

Childhood sexual exploration can be between *same gender* or between *boys* and *girls*. Statistically there are no significant trends. When college students were asked about "showing their privates" to others, it was sometimes with a child of the same gender and sometimes with the other gender. The same was true of "touching the private parts" of other children. Generally, the gender a person prefers to engage in sex with becomes important around puberty. Early childhood exploration is more a matter of who your friends are, who is willing, and who is there when the situation is ripe for experimentation.

Boys and Girls Are Both Curious

There are few differences between the sexual behaviors of young boys and girls. There are many books right now describing male and female adult sexuality as very different—such as John Gray's *Men are from Mars and Women Are from Venus*. In young children's sexual behaviors, however, there aren't so many differences. In fact little girls seems to engage in about as much sexual behavior as boys. Perhaps male sexuality is more visible than female sexuality, or perhaps socialization has more to do with men's and women's sexuality as they traverse adolescence and young adulthood.

We generally think of adult men as being more sexually oriented than women. It's interesting that in the college student study there were no significant differences between males and females in their sexual behaviors or in their feelings when engaging in the sexual behaviors. For instance, whether alone or with one other child, boys were more likely to behave in a sexual manner, but not significantly more than the girls. Overall 60% of the students said they engaged in solitary sexual behaviors. Of this 63% were boys and 55% were girls. When engaging with one other child overall 57% said they did this. Of this number 63% were boys and 56% were girls. Overall 20% of the students said they engaged in sexual behaviors with at least two or more children. Of this number 25% were males and 16% were females.

Fourteen percent of the students said they were coerced into sexual behaviors. Of the students who said they were coerced 18% were males while 12% were females. We often think of boys being more aggressive when it comes to most behaviors and sexual behaviors would probably be the same. In the college sample it was 7% of the sample who coerced others into sexual behaviors. Of this number 9% were males and 4% were females. Neither the victimization or coercion of other children was statistically different for males and females.

Pleasure

Many children experience *pleasant sensations* if they touch their own genitals, some children may experience sexual arousal, and some will experience orgasm. At birth and in utero children have all of the sexual apparatus necessary for adult sexual behavior. Infants' vaginas can lubricate, boys can have erections, the clitoris can be stimulated, children can have orgasms, the fallopian tubes are present, and the eggs are all stored and ready to be released at puberty when menstruation begins.

Although all of the apparatus is present most children don't experience sexual orgasms and pleasure similar to that experienced by adults until puberty. With puberty and the major influx of the sexual hormones the body and mind are more driven toward genital contact and erotic pleasure. Children do experience pleasant sensations when their genitals are stimulated but this isn't the same as the orgasmic pleasure, which is more pervasive after puberty.

Thirty-two percent of the mental health and child welfare professionals described feeling "pleasant body sensations" when engaging in sexual behaviors between the ages of eleven to twelve, 27% felt "pleasant body sensations" between ages six to ten. When asked if they felt "sexually stimulated as an adult might feel," 21% did when they were eleven to twelve, 9% when they were six to ten. The college students said they felt more "sexually stimulated as an adult might feel" when engaging in sexual behaviors alone (22%) than when engaging in sexual behaviors with other children (17%).

Only 17% of the students said they had masturbated to orgasm when they were between eleven to twelve years of age, 4% said they did this between the ages of six to ten. More girls (17%) than boys (8%) masturbated to orgasm when twelve and younger. This may be due to girls going through puberty earlier. Orgasm is a far more frequent experience in postpubertal children.

Secrecy

If children are discovered in normal sex play and instructed to stop, the sexual behavior will probably *diminish* or *cease, at least in the sight of adults*, but may arise again during another period of their sexual development. Infants and toddlers show more of their sexual behaviors than when they get to preschool and kindergarten. Adults generally tell children not to do such things as touch their genitals or the private parts of others. Thus the children stop doing it in front of the adults.

Swearing is a good example. Young children around four and five often begin to say words such as "shit." You may react very negatively to your child saying these things—most adults do. So your child may learn to swear in private with their friends or even stop for a while. There are probably very few children who go through their elementary school years without experimenting with lots of "bad" words.

When children become old enough to understand adults' reactions to sexual exploration, secrecy becomes the hallmark of sexual behavior. When asked whether any adult knew about their sexual experiences with other children around the time they engaged in them, 90% of the college students said "no." When asked, "Did you tell anyone about your sexual behaviors?", 84% of college students said "no."

Coercion

An important aspect of childhood sexual exploration is that it is usually *without pressure*. "I'll show you mine, if you show me yours" is a time-honored phrase. It implies that one child is asking another to explore with him or her. Another phrase is "I'll be your best friend if you'll show me your pee-pee." This implies that the child asking will like the other child more if he or she complies with the request. Between two friends this is not of concern. One child might feel slightly pressured to engage in the behavior, but he or she would also know that the threat probably wouldn't come true for long. A friend would also know that they could refuse to continue if he or she wanted to stop. Friends partake in this type of mild coercion regularly, in the sexual realm and outside of it.

For instance, if a child wants to liberate some of his mother's freshly baked cookies and wants his friend to go with him he might threaten, "If you don't come with me, I won't play with you ever again," or, "If you don't come with me, I won't give you any. I'll eat them all myself."

If a child is using the same types of "threats" with children who have no friends or desperately want to be that particular child's friend but is always rebuffed, these statements can feel very threatening. A vulnerable child may acquiesce out of fear of losing an opportunity for friendship. This is *not* in the realm of natural and healthy play.

When describing sexual encounters among two or more children, the college students described some of their coercive techniques. At the top of the list were teasing (such as calling the other child a chicken), then begging, bribery, trickery, physical force, verbal threats, and physical pain. The average age at which these experiences occurred was nine years old. Clearly the methods used moved to more aggressive coercion that any child might have been able to withstand whether or not the other child was a friend.

Fourteen percent of the students said they had been tricked, bribed, threatened, forced, or otherwise coerced into sexual behaviors by someone twelve or younger when they were twelve or younger. Seven percent said they had bribed, teased, threatened, physically forced, or otherwise coerced another child twelve or younger to engage in sexual behaviors with them when they were twelve or younger.

Important Points to Consider about Your Child's Sexual Behaviors

There are some points about childhood sexuality that are important for you to consider as you are understanding your child's sexuality.

- *Most behaviors related to sex and sexuality in young children are natural and expectable.* Understanding sexuality is an important area of your growing child's expanding knowledge. Sexual exploration and sexual play are a natural part of your child's development. Accept this and help him or her feel comfortable while also knowing the limits.

- *Your own childhood sexual experiences may have been quite different than your child's.* It's not advisable to use your own childhood experience as the norm for sexual experience. When you do this you may believe that your own experience was the norm. This may not be true at all. If you didn't engage with other children in any sexual behavior, you may think it's not normal to do so. If you didn't talk to other children about their sexual behaviors as a child, you didn't know what other children were doing. If you engaged in some solitary sexual behavior and felt bad about it, you may carry this over to your children. If you were caught and scolded for sexually experimenting, you may feel guilty and bad for the behavior. It's best to look at the facts presented throughout this book and make your assessments based on a wider data pool.

  Things have changed. Speaking with other parents and caregivers who have children of similar ages is helpful in determining what is natural and healthy. There is a great deal more sexual stimulation in our culture today, and children have a greater knowledge about sexual behaviors than in previous generations. Your experience was shaped by your culture, your parents, your siblings, the religion in which you were raised, where you lived, as well as other things. These factors are different for your child. Be current.

- *Don't confuse your own adult sexual feelings, fantasies, and behavior with those of children.* Most prepubertal children do not experience sexual arousal and sexual pleasure, but some do. In prepubertal children, the sexual activity generally doesn't represent the desire for sexual gratification as much as exploration of their bodies, other's bodies, and gender roles. Children describe different sensations related to the sexual exploration. Some are sexually arousing and pleasurable; others describe them as weird or funny; others say they are exciting, as in doing something forbidden. Some children whose sexual development has been interfered with by adults describe their genital sensations as "uncomfortable," "icky," "confusing," or "scary."

  Even though children's sexual behaviors may look like adult sexual behaviors, it generally isn't experienced with the erotic and sensual components. This is important information to consider as some adults are disgusted thinking a child is engaging in adult sexual behaviors with the same thoughts and feelings as themselves and then treat the children as disgusting, weird, lost to Satan, and so on.

- *The relationships we have as we grow up are fundamental to our healthy development.* The best foundation for healthy adult relationships is secure attachments to adults and family as your children grow up. A secure relationship or attachment is one in which your relationship to your child is consistent, caring, reliable, and focused on the needs of your child rather than your own. If a child feels insecure in his or her relationships with adults, this will make it more difficult for them to feel secure in adult relationships and to provide this feeling for their children.

    For example, if adults in a child's life have sexualized relationships with him or her, or the child has only seen failed relationships that were sexualized, permissive, aggressive, hurtful, and unfulfilling, this will impact a child's view of the role that sex plays in adult relationships.

- *As we have learned more about the sexual abuse of children, sexual behavior between children sometimes causes too much concern.* What starts out as two children exploring each other's genitals can end up with one or both being interviewed by child protective services and/or the police due to concern that they have been sexually abused. While caution is always necessary, there are many clues to children being sexually abused and sexual behavior is only one of them.

    Sexual behaviors that are indicators of sexual abuse by an adult or an adolescent rarely fit the pattern of natural and healthy sexual development described in this chapter. There are no childhood sexual behaviors that have been seen only by mothers of sexually abused children. There is no single behavior that indicates sexual abuse. See chapter 3 for the characteristics of sexual behaviors that increase the concern that a child has been sexually abused in a hands-on manner or has been exposed to too much adolescent or adult sexuality.

CHAPTER 3

Characteristics of Problematic Sexual Behaviors During Childhood

In previous chapters I have described natural and healthy sexual behaviors of children. In this chapter I will describe characteristics of children's sexual behaviors that can alert you to possible problems with your child's sexual development.

Assessing Your Child's Behavior

If your child's sexual behavior can be described by several of the following characteristics, and your parental intervention hasn't curtailed the behavior, and you cannot find a reasonable and healthy explanation for this, your child should be evaluated by a *qualified professional*. Find a professional who is knowledgeable about child sexuality or child abuse. You may also need to have your child medically examined.

There are many reasons that can contribute to a child's sexual development getting confused. Most people think it is always hands-on sexual abuse. This isn't true. Factors that can contribute to a child engaging in problematic sexual behaviors are discussed in chapter 4. It will be important for you to not jump to any conclusions about your child as you read. The characteristics toward the beginning of the list are less worrisome than the characteristics toward the end of the list.

1. *The children engaged in the sexual behaviors do not have an ongoing mutual play relationship.* Sexual play between children is an extension of regular play behavior. Just as children prefer to play with children with whom they get along, this is the same with sexual play. As most children are very aware of taboos on sexual play in the open, they pick friends who will keep the secret.

    Haugaard's (1988) research regarding children involved in sexual play indicates that for boys 82% of the time the other child is a friend (girls 79%); 10% of the time the other child is an acquaintance (girls 10%); 1% of the time a stranger (girls 1%); and 8% of the time a relative (girls 12%).

    Finkelhor's data (1973) indicate that experiences with friends are clearly more frequent than experiences with siblings. While not all sexual experiences with siblings are negative there is a higher likelihood that a positive experience will be with a friend.

2. *Sexual behaviors that are engaged in by children of different ages or developmental levels* Unless there are no similar-age children in the neighborhood, most children select playmates of the same age. Yet, developmentally delayed children may choose to play with younger children because their developmental level is more similar. Children with poor social skills may also play with younger children.

    It's important to assess the availability of peer-age friends, developmental level, and the previous relationship between the children to determine if sexual behaviors among children of different ages are problematic. In general, the wider the age difference, the greater the concern.

    Research indicates that the average difference in age between children who engage in sex play is approximately four to eight months (Haugaard 1988). Finkelhor's (1973) study shows that the greater the age difference between the children the more negative the reaction to the sexual experience. The most positive experiences for both boys and girls was when the age difference was less than a year. The most negative experiences for girls was when the sexual experience was with someone five or more years older.

3. *Sexual behaviors that are out of balance with other aspects of the child's life and interests.* Children are interested in every aspect of their environment from the sun rising to how babies are made. While children may explore some aspects of their world more extensively at certain periods of their young lives, their interests are generally broad and intermittent.

   Children's sexual behavior follows the same pattern. At one period they may be interested in learning about sexuality and another time about how the dishwasher works or what makes Mommy mad. Many fluctuations occur in a day, a week, and a month. But, when a child is preoccupied with sexuality, this raises concern. If a child prefers to masturbate rather than participate in regular childhood activities, this raises concern.

4. *Children who seem to have too much knowledge about sexuality and behave in ways more consistent with adult sexual expression.* As children develop, they acquire knowledge about sex and sexuality from television, movies, videos, magazines, their parents, relatives, school, and other children. Knowledge gathered in these time-honored ways is generally assimilated, without disruption, into a child's developing understanding of sex and sexuality; this translates into additional natural and healthy sexual interest. When children have been overexposed to explicit adult sexuality, or have been sexually misused, they may engage in or talk about sexual behaviors that are beyond age-appropriate sexual knowledge and interest.

5. *Sexual behaviors that are significantly different than those of other same-age children.* The frequency and type of children's sexual behaviors depend, to a certain extent, on the environment (home, neighborhood, culture, religion) in which they have been raised, their parent's attitudes and actions related to sex and sexuality, and their peers' behaviors. If a child's sexual behavior stands out among his or her neighborhood peers, this raises concern. Teachers from schools who serve neighborhood populations are very good resources to consult to evaluate whether or not a child's sexual behaviors are similar to his or her peers.

6. *Sexual behaviors that continue in spite of consistent and clear requests to stop.* While adults may be inconsistent regarding other behaviors and children may persist in engaging in them, most children learn very quickly that there's a strong taboo on openly sexual behavior. Yet while most adults are consistent about telling children to stop, some aren't. Inconsistent messages regarding sexual behavior may increase, or not decrease, a child's sexual behaviors. For example, if you think it's cute when your child runs around the house naked but punish your child sometimes, it may be hard for him or her to learn the rules.

Children's sexual behaviors that continue in the view of adults, despite consistent requests to stop or even punishment, may be a conscious or unconscious method of indicating that they need help. When children "cry for help," they may persist in the behavior until adults pay heed, discover, and/or change the causes of the sexual behavior. Sometimes children who are being sexually abused signal the abuse by engaging in persistent sexual behaviors.

Certain children have learned to "space out" in times of stress. While they're spaced out, they may engage in sexual behavior, which itself is another way to decrease their anxiety. If this is happening, the child may be unaware of the sexual behaviors he or she is doing. Because the child's response to stress is to space out and engage in sexual behaviors, it may happen in spite of consistent requests to stop. Children who space out need help to stay present and cope with their feelings and thoughts that create the anxiety. They need the help of adults who can help figure out what causes them to space out.

7. *Children who appear unable to stop themselves from participating in sexual activities.* Some children appear to feel driven to engage in sexual behaviors even though they'll be punished or admonished. Typically, this type of sexual behavior is in response to things that go on around them or feelings that reawaken memories which are traumatic, painful, overly stimulating, or of which they can't make sense. The child may respond by masturbating or engaging in other sexual experimentation behaviors alone or with children or adults. Hiding the sexual behaviors or finding friends to engage in the behaviors in private, may not be possible for these children. Sexual behavior that is driven by anxiety, guilt, or fear often doesn't respond to normal limit setting. The sexual

behavior is a way of coping with overwhelming feelings. This type of sexual behavior may not be within the full conscious control of the child.

Recent research on brain development is suggesting a relationship between early stress and neurobiological changes in the brain. It's possible that children raised in chaotic environments who experience a wide range of early experiences in which sex is paired with anger, hurt, or overstimulation may have changes in their brain chemistry, altering their experience of sex and sexuality as they grow up.

Some children may have psychiatric disturbances such as obsessive-compulsive disorder that cause them to partake in repetitive behaviors. These could be sexual as well as other kinds of rituals. Some children may have urinary tract or yeast infections that cause chronic itching or sensations, which look like sexual touching.

8. *Children's sexual behaviors that elicit complaints from other children and/or adversely affect other children.* Generally, children complain when something is annoying or discomforting to them. When a young child complains about another child's sexual behaviors, it's an indication that the behavior is upsetting to the child and should be taken seriously. In natural and healthy sexual play both children agree directly or indirectly not to tell and are involved in the behavior willingly. It's quite unlikely that either would tell on the other; therefore, if one child is telling, this is a cause for concern.

Alternatively, on school playgrounds elementary school boys and girls run after one another discovering who has the most "cooties." When the children are equal in age, developmental status, and are having fun together, these complaints can be a spirited age-appropriate interchange that need only be monitored to see that it remains fun and noncoercive.

9. *Children's sexual behaviors that are directed at adults who feel uncomfortable receiving them.* Children hug adults and give them kisses. These are generally spontaneous reflections of caring or because they have been told to kiss the adult (usually a relative) by a parent. When a child continues to touch an adult in a manner more like adult-adult sexual contact, offer themselves as sexual objects, or solicit sexual touch from adults, this may be an indication that someone is

teaching the child to engage in age-inappropriate sexual contact. When children are sexually abused, the abuse may take the form of teaching the child to sexually pleasure the adult. Young children may generalize this to their contact with other adults. If children are doing this, it will be important to find out how the child is learning to engage in this type of physical contact. Child protective services can be called if there is a suspicion of child abuse.

It's important that children who engage in this type of physical contact be assisted to learn natural and healthy ways to touch others. Because touch is essential for healthy development it's important that all children have physical contact with others. In some cases a child might be punished by allowing no physical contact. This is contraindicated as it may push the child to seek out physical contact with people who will take advantage of him or her.

It's best to model healthy physical contact and teach the child while practicing with him or her. It will also be helpful to find lots of ways to have physical contact. Examples are: hot hands (the game); tag; football; sparring; reading a book with someone; combing or cutting hair; applying a bandage or a brace; a pat on the back or shoulder; tussle of the child's hair; hugs; sideways hug; shaking hands; and so on.

It is important to decrease sexualized contact between a child and adult because this may be seen by a sex offender. Sex offenders may take advantage of a child who already engages in sexualized behavior. If a sex offender believes a child has been sexually abused by observing age-inappropriate contact with adults, he or she may target the child as an easy victim.

10. *Children (four years and older) who do not understand their rights or the rights of others in relation to sexual contact.* Most parents teach their children by their own behavior about emotional, physical, and sexual privacy. Generally, school-age children have developed an awareness of their own and others' personal space. If children are brought up in homes where their personal boundaries are violated, such as in emotional, sexual and/or physical abuse or intrusiveness, they may not learn the unwritten rules regarding personal space violations

11. *Sexual behaviors that progress in frequency, intensity, or intrusiveness over time.* When sexual behavior in young children is

natural and healthy, the frequency is generally moderate, the behaviors occur sporadically and mostly occur outside the vision and knowledge of others. As most children grow up there's an increase in the sexual behaviors and they transition from looking to touching. But by elementary school age, children increasingly hide their sexual behaviors from adults. If adults know a lot about the child's sexual behaviors, this may be because either the children are interfering with other children and being reported, they don't understand healthy contact, or they're unable to contain the sexual behaviors. This is uncommon and raises concern.

12. *When fear, anxiety, deep shame, or intense guilt is associated with the sexual behaviors.* Children's feelings regarding sexuality are generally lighthearted, spontaneous, giggly, or silly. In some cases, if a child has been caught engaging in sexual behaviors, the adult's response may have generated embarrassed or guilty feelings in the child. Yet, these feelings are qualitatively different than the deep shame, intense guilt, fear, or anxiety of a child who has been fooled, coerced, bribed, or threatened into sexual behaviors, or overexposed to adult sexuality, particularly sexuality paired with aggressive feelings or actions.

13. *Children who engage in extensive, persistent mutually agreed upon adult-type sexual behaviors with other children.* Children generally engage in a variety of spontaneous and sporadic sexual behaviors with other children for purposes of exploration and the satisfaction of curiosity. Some children who feel alone in the world may turn to other children to decrease their loneliness. These children often do not see adults as sources of emotional warmth and caring. If the children have been prematurely sexualized and/or taught that sex equals caring, they may try to use sex as a way to cope with their loneliness. (See page 86.)

14. *Children who manually stimulate or have oral or genital contact with animals.* Children in urban and suburban areas rarely have contact with the genitalia of animals. Children on farms might have some sexual contact with animals but it is limited. Children who engage in repeated sexualized behaviors with animals or who harm animals raise concern.

15. *Children sexualize nonsexual things, or interactions with others, or relationships.* For example, the child imagines "she wants to be my girlfriend," or "he is thinking about doing sex"

without any observable basis for thinking this. The child sees everyday objects as sexual or people as sexual objects.

16. *Sexual behaviors that cause physical or emotional pain or discomfort to self or others.* Children who engage in any behaviors, including sexual behaviors, which induce pain or discomfort to themselves or others, cause concern.

17. *Children who use sex to hurt others.* When sex and pain, sex and disappointment, sex and hurt, sex and jealousy, or sex and other negative emotions and experiences have been paired, the children may use sex as a weapon. Angry sexual language and gestures as well as sexual touching becomes a way to get back at people. This can be in much the same way as it has been used against them.

18. *When verbal and/or physical expressions of anger precede, follow, or accompany the sexual behavior.* In healthy development, sexual expression and exploration is accompanied by positive emotions. Verbal or physical aggression that accompanies children's sexual behaviors is a learned response to sexuality. In general, children who repeat this behavior have witnessed repeated instances in which verbally and/or physically aggressive behavior has occurred, in the context of sex. Children may have witnessed their parents or other adults hitting one another when fighting about sexual matters. Some children may have witnessed a parent being sexually misused. Some parents use highly sexual words when verbally assaulting their partners.

Children who have been sexually abused may feel anger and suspicion about all sexual expression. When children associate negative and hostile emotions with sexual behavior, this may be their response to having been coerced, forced, bribed, fooled, manipulated, or threatened into sexual contact or they may be aware of this happening to someone else. When verbal or physical expressions of anger are paired with the child's sexual expression, this is cause for great concern.

When children use bad language it's generally with each other and out of the earshot of adults. Whereas many parents disapprove of this, it's not uncommon for children eight years and older. The use of sexual words combined with violence is not common and is a cause for concern. Pairing sex with violence in words, actions, or deeds is always a cause for concern. Parents need to be aware that children model the behavior of those around them. If parents, friends, or people in the neighborhood are using this type of language, children may well be following in their footsteps.

19. *Children who use distorted logic to justify their sexual actions.* ("She didn't say 'no.'") When caught doing something wrong, children often try to make an excuse. But when young children make excuses about their sexual behaviors that disregard others' rights or deny responsibility for their troublesome sexual behaviors, this raises concern. For instance, a child who says he was grabbing at a girl's bottom because she had on a short skirt, or the girl who said she was grabbing at the penis of a boy because "all boys like sex stuff"—these are signs of a child using distorted logic.

    This type of behavior in children may be a reflection of modeling behavior seen and heard in the nuclear or extended family. The media's portrayal of sexual stereotypes and violations of others' personal rights as acceptable may encourage this behavior as well.

20. *When coercion, force, bribery, manipulation, or threats are associated with sexual behaviors.* Healthy sexual exploration may include teasing or daring; unhealthy sexual expression involves the use of emotional or physical force or coercion to involve another child in sexual behavior. Children who engage in coercive sexual behavior generally target a child who is emotionally or physically vulnerable. Although infrequent in young children, groups of children may coerce one or more children into doing a sexual behavior.

After reading about the characteristics of children's sexual behaviors that raise concern, you may have found that your child does some. Make sure you have read about healthy sexuality and gauged your child's behavior from that point of view also. Look for the balance of healthy and problematic in your child's behavior. Since parents know their children better than anyone else, you will want to decide if the problematic characteristics you see in your child's behavior need to be modified and how you want to do it. If you have a spouse or partner, you should decide together.

Chapter 11 talks about communication between parents and children. It gives both you and your child good ideas about how to talk to each other. Chapter 6 discusses a range of sexual behaviors in children. You can see if you can place your child in any one these groups. If your child fits in the "sexually-reactive" group you may want to use chapter 7 on decreasing problematic sexual behaviors in young children. If your child fits in any of the other groups, you'll need professional assistance.

If you decide you need help, you can contact your pediatrician or a licensed mental health professional with experience in child development, child sexuality, or child sexual abuse. He or she will help guide you to modify your child's problematic sexual behavior. If your pediatrician does not know of qualified mental health professionals, you can call your local outpatient mental health agency, the department of mental health, the department of child protective services, your priest or minister, your child's school counselor, or ask your local hospital mental health department.

Pay Attention—But Don't Jump to Conclusions

Be careful not to be too hasty in your assessment. The following stories illustrate how you can become immediately apprehensive and, if not careful, could jump to the wrong conclusion. Children explore their bodies and other children's bodies. It's important not to conclude that your child has been molested or that your child is engaging in problematic sexual behaviors. *Be calm. Gather information.* Don't lead your child into saying something that may not be true. And don't make your child feel guilty. Slowly gather information without making anything a big issue. Children often stop talking when they think they've done something wrong or when they see you getting anxious or upset.

Deep Space Exploration

At four Arlyne was into everything. She fired questions nonstop at anyone who would listen. The sun and the moon and the stars were her current interest. Her parents were even thinking of inviting a space scientist friend of theirs over to answer her questions. She had far outstripped their knowledge base.

Arlyne's Aunt Marie was helping bathe her one morning. As Marie was helping her dry herself, Arlyne sat down on the floor and spread her legs. "Look, look, there's a hole down there." Excitedly, she put her finger in her vaginal opening. Aunt Marie, a social worker, immediately panicked. She tried to keep calm, and she said, "You're right, there is a hole down there."

Arlyne, while bending her body as only young children can do, took her finger out of her vaginal opening and tried to look in "Wow, it goes in real far." Aunt Marie remained calm. Then Arlyne said, "Things go in there?" Marie began to rapidly think of possible suspects who could have had access to her niece. She could feel her fear rising.

"God," she thought, "I've done everything to protect children in the community against sex offenders and someone has gotten to my niece. Who could it be?" Marie tried to think of every man who could have inappropriately touched Arlyne. Then, in a panic, she also thought of all of the women who might have inappropriately touched her. She realized she needed to calm herself and get back to her niece.

Marie became aware of how different this situation was from all of the other children she had interviewed over the last twenty years. She couldn't stay dispassionate. She was having trouble getting enough distance between her feelings and the situation with her niece to even sound calm. All Marie really wanted to say to Arlyne was, "Has anyone touched your hole?" But she knew she had to stick with open-ended, nonspecific questions. She couldn't lead her in any particular direction. Marie didn't want to say anything that might confuse an investigation, if there turned out to be a legitimate suspicion of abuse.

Arlyne startled Marie even further by stating, "Something must go in this hole 'cause it's so deep." "What kind of things might go in that hole?" asked Marie. Arlyne brightened up and said, "You know." Aunt Marie felt her heart racing, but didn't want to ask direct questions. Instead she asked Arlyne, "You're so smart, you tell me." Arlyne said, "Mommy uses them. Do you put stuff in your hole Aunt Marie?"

Marie began to think Arlyne was talking about tampons but still tried to keep the questions open-ended and not goal-directed. She said, "What stuff do you mean?" "That long thing. It fits right in there." Marie began to feel she was being tortured and the torturer was four! "A long thing," Marie said. "Yes, you know," responded Arlyne. Feeling brave, Marie asked, "Can you show me?"

Arlyne jumped up and went to the closet and got a box of tampons. She said, "Mommy puts these in. I tried but I can't get it in. Can you help me?" Relief came over Marie. Apparently, Arlyne had seen her mother inserting tampons. This explained her interest in her "hole." Aunt Marie explained that tampons are for grown-ups and not children. Arlyne wanted to know why. Emotionally spent, Marie told her to ask her mother. Aunt Marie wasn't sure that she ever wanted to bathe Arlyne again!

In Handcuffs at Eight

The need for careful and thorough evaluation of children referred for problem sexual behaviors is evident in the case of eight-year-old Ian, who was referred for evaluation after a long and traumatic day. Ian had been taken from his apartment in handcuffs and put into a police squad car as the neighbors watched. Phoned by the police, Ian's parents met him at the police station. The allegation against the third-grader was sexual assault.

Earlier that day, the apartment manager's two young daughters (ages four and five) came to their mother and announced that Ian had pulled down their pants and tried to touch their private parts. The manager immediately phoned the police, who responded by transporting Ian to the police station. After questioning Ian and his parents, in lieu of immediately filing charges, the police referred the family for an evaluation at a center with special expertise in treating children who molest other children. The parents followed up by scheduling an appointment immediately.

As soon as Ian's parents arrived, they presented an immediate contrast to the fragmented and multiproblem families of children who molest. Ian's mother and father both attended the session with Ian and instead of being hostile or denying the allegations, made it clear that they took the incident with the neighbor children seriously and that they were concerned about their son. Their intake information revealed a stable family history. Ian's parents had been married for eighteen years. They also had an older son, a sixteen-year-old who was a good student. Both parents had worked for the same company for over ten years. There was no history of drugs, alcohol, physical or sexual abuse, or major family disruption.

Up until his arrest, Ian's history also showed positive stability and achievement. He was doing fine academically, was a Little League player, and had many friends. The assessment instruments filled out by Ian's parents and teacher indicated no significant behavioral problems. His parents filled out the *Child Sexual Behavior Checklist* (Johnson 1996) which indicated sexual behaviors within normal limits. All questions related to abuse, abandonment, neglect, or a highly sexually charged family atmosphere were met with negative responses.

In the interview with Ian alone, the eight-year-old quietly told the therapist that he knew what he had done was wrong and that he was sorry. He explained that his motive in approaching the girls was curiosity. Alone in the apartment all day during summer vacation, there was little to do. "And I really did wonder," Eddie said, "what girls look like." Then he added, "I hope I didn't scare them."

The two little girls were interviewed the following day, and the therapist asked them if they were afraid of Eddie. "No way!" they insisted, giggling. Further questioning revealed that Eddie didn't play with them regularly, only in the swimming pool. When the girls went swimming he would go also because the manager acted as a lifeguard. He was only allowed out of his apartment when his parents were at work to swim and he could only swim when there was a lifeguard. He'd never tried anything sexual with the girls before and had always gotten along with them.

On the other hand, Ian's sexual behavior with the children had clearly been inappropriate. He'd not only asked to "look" but had pulled down both the children's pants and tried to touch their private parts without their permission or mutual agreement. His behavior caused special concern because the girls were considerably younger than he and not regular playmates who engaged in other mutually enjoyable activities. The girls indicated, however, that Ian stopped immediately when they said, "No!" and he hadn't threatened, bribed, or tried to stop them from running after their mother who'd momentarily gone into the laundry room.

After assessing Ian, the evaluator felt that his behavior was of concern and should be monitored, but that it didn't go far beyond the curiosity of other children. If Ian had had regular same-age playmates, he would've been experimenting with them.

After discussions with Ian and his parents about natural and healthy sexual behavior in children and feeling confident that the family understood what had happened, they were provided with materials regarding sexuality. The evaluator encouraged Ian and his family to have open discussions regarding sexual issues. The evaluator also pointed out that Ian needed a more structured schedule and planned activities. Eight-year-olds may well get into mischief if left alone all day in an apartment complex without supervision or playmates their own age. His parents agreed and enrolled him in a local day camp for summer and an afternoon day care program for the school year.

Finally, the interviewing therapist gave Ian's parents a list of problematic sexual behaviors of children and other behaviors that occur in children who have problems in the area of sexuality. "Call me if Ian starts doing things on this list," the therapist urged. "Let's set an appointment for two months from now just to see how things are going for Ian. Then we'll be in phone contact on a six month basis or as needed."

All future contacts with Ian and his family indicated no further sexual problems. He has subsequently completed puberty and started dating. His behavior with girls is respectful. At seventeen he has engaged in kissing and fondling but says that he doesn't plan to have sexual intercourse until he is in a serious, committed relationship.

The Child with No Boundaries

When children engage in advanced sexual behaviors it's very confusing to the adults. Has the child been sexually abused? Is the child a danger to other children? Is the child molesting other children? These questions need to be considered very carefully. It is important not to jump to conclusions.

With rancor in her voice a preschool principal phoned one morning and asked for an evaluation of a five-year-old boy engaging in what she described as "molesting behavior." She told James' parents that he could no longer attend her school unless he was supervised by his mother or a relative. There had been two events of sexual behavior at the school between James and another child and several heated discussions with Jana, James' mother. The mother of the other child had called a lawyer who had subsequently called the principal.

James' mother refused to supervise James saying it was the school's responsibility. She also refused to remove him from the school because she didn't want his life disrupted or to make him feel he'd done something wrong. The principal had demanded an evaluation of James by a specialist with recommendations regarding how to handle the situation.

Loud arguing in the evaluator's waiting room between James' recently divorced parents signaled problems from the start. During the initial interview, Jana accused her ex-husband, Drew, James' father, of not doing anything for her son, requiring her to carry the entire burden. The animosity between the parents was fierce. It appeared that Jana felt helpless and in need of support but her relentless attacks on the school, the teacher, the principal, her ex-husband, and eventually the evaluator made it hard to find acceptable ways to intervene to help her, her husband, and James.

After filling out the *Child Sexual Behavior Checklist* (Johnson 1996), a list of 150 children's sexual behaviors related to sex and sexuality, and the *Child Behavior Checklist* (Acherbach 1983), it became apparent that James was engaging in many sexualized behaviors with other children outside of school in addition to the behaviors at school. While all of the sexualized behaviors with other children were consensual, there was more sexual contact than is generally expected, or at least, than adults would generally know about.

There were three instances in the summer when James was found with different friends, girls and boys, with their pants down exploring each other's genitals. One time James was found with a boy in James' room with the door open, another time James and a girl were discovered in his room again with the door open. The third time the children were found in James' closet with the door closed, yet the door to his bedroom was open. The first two incidents were at his mother's house, the third at his father's house.

One of the incidents at school involved James and his friend putting their mouths on each other's naked penis. This behavior happened in the classroom under a table they had made into a tent by covering it with a blanket. They were discovered because they were giggling loudly. In another previous incident at school, James was in the bathroom with the same boy and both had their pants down. Each boy was moving his body to make their penis wiggle. Other behaviors related to sex and sexuality occurred at James' mother's house where he fondled himself watching television while naked. James was also likely to open the front door naked if someone knocked or go outside naked if he felt like it.

From the *Child Behavior Checklist* (Acherbach 1983), it was apparent that James was significantly more disruptive and disobedient at his mother's house than at his father's. He was often defiant, and would sometimes lie or take others' things. The teacher described James' behavior as generally kind, but often disobedient. He got along well with most of the children, was bright and enthusiastic, but didn't follow directions that he didn't want to follow. James behaved well when his father picked him up from school. But when his mother came to pick James up he was often disruptive and argumentative unless she promised to take him to get ice cream or some other special treat. She would initially try to passively cajole him to comply but she would eventually get angry and upset with his misbehavior and pull him out of the school.

James entered the evaluator's room on his first visit curious to explore all of it. He went from toy to toy picking things up and looking at them only to drop them on the floor or leave them askew. He was polite but seemed not to notice the evaluator until he was finished with his exploration. For a five-year-old bright, enthusiastic boy this didn't seem remarkable although the general disorder he made seemed a bit curious. When asked to draw his family doing something he drew a picture of him and his father playing baseball in his father's backyard. When asked about his mother, he took another sheet and drew her by herself.

Because of the frequency of James' known behaviors related to sex and sexuality there was concern that someone was engaging James in sexual behaviors or that he was somehow watching adults or adolescents engaged in sexual behavior in real life, in movies, or on videos. After two sessions with James in which he was open to answering questions, it appeared that there had been no questionable sexual contact between James and anyone else other than the children. Nor was there any exposure to adult or adolescent sexuality or sexual material in print, movies, TV, or videos. James didn't have any knowledge about sex or sexuality that appeared too advanced for his age nor did he evidence any undue concerns about any aspects of his life.

James' descriptions of his morning and evening routines at his mother's house indicated arguments over bedtime and eating but nothing sexualized or aggressive. His description of life at his father's also seemed orderly with standard parent-child interactions.

As most children of divorced parents, James talked about wishing his mother and father would get married again. He would often hear them arguing about money while they all were still living together. James' descriptions of his parents' interactions was reminiscent of their argument in the principal's waiting room. While it was clear that James had been privy to too much of his parents arguing, the language was not laced with vituperative comments using salacious and sexual terms. No violence was evidenced in James' recreation of the scenes and no sexual behavior by the parents or anyone else in either home was evident.

When young children engage in dangerous, aggressive, or forced sexual behavior their home environment generally is characterized by some or all of the following: drugs, alcohol, people coming in and out randomly, unacceptable sexual behaviors in front of the children, the pairing of sex and aggression, physical battering between adults, emotional or physical abuse or other disordered and stress-producing events. These cause children's emotional and sexual development to become disorganized and take a developmentally unexpected trajectory.

It emerged from the evaluation that James' mother was bathing with James, that nudity was practiced fairly regularly at her house, and that she didn't curtail James from fondling his genitals when he was undressed on the living room sofa. The genital fondling occurred when he watched morning cartoons or, on some occasions, in the evening.

James' father no longer allowed James to do this at his house but acknowledged that this did occur when he lived with the family and that nudity was common. He said he usually dressed now that James was getting older and very curious about his body. However, he still showered with James occasionally because it was faster than trying to get James to take a bath. He acknowledged that James showed considerable interest in his penis and he'd had to tell him he could not touch it as he frequently requested. Both parents agreed that James had enormous curiosity about sex, that sexuality and the body were on the top of his list of interests since the beginning of the summer.

Jana insisted that her whole family had always been nude at home and that her parents had given her a good sense about her body. She planned to give that to James. She felt it was acceptable for James to fondle himself on the sofa in the living room, regardless of her walking in and out of the room. She also did not see a problem with James going outside naked in the yard at his age. She didn't want him to think naked bodies were bad or that sex was bad.

When James came to a session accompanied by his mother and aunt, the evaluator found support for her developing hypothesis that James' sexual behavior was a reflection of the open atmosphere about nudity, bodies, and sexuality in his mother's home, James' high level of sexual interest, and his parent's ineffective parenting skills. James' aunt had accompanied Jana and James to the session as Jana felt there was no way she could have even a brief uninterrupted talk with the evaluator unless James had someone with whom to play.

Even with the aunt to care for him, James disrupted the session between the evaluator and Jana five times in the fifteen minutes they were together. Each time Jana was accepting of the interruption and then grew frustrated by James not leaving after his questions were answered. Jana appeared to have no parenting tactics with James between "please behave" and complete frustration.

Apparently James wasn't only being given great leeway regarding nudity and sexuality but was also not being asked to conform to any boundaries regarding any of his behaviors. James didn't know what was acceptable and unacceptable behavior and he was not being provided adequate guidance regarding restraining his behavior. James' mother didn't understand that her lack of discipline was causing him to balk at the few admonitions she did give him. James did not respect or apparently want to be with her except when she was "nice," which meant her placing no restrictions on his behavior. He felt much closer to his father and was unable to sort out his mother's inconsistent messages. This proved too difficult for a five-year-old to understand.

At school and at his father's home, this contributed to James only conforming when the boundaries were made very clear, when he was under high supervision, and when there was an imminent punishment. Just as he wasn't conforming to the classroom rules, likewise he was not conforming to the expectations of others around sexual behaviors. A significant problem for James was that he didn't know the norms around sexual behaviors since he hadn't been given clear guidelines.

It was interesting that when he engaged in the genital showing and touching at his father's house, James knew to go in the closet but still didn't close the door to his room. At his mother's house he didn't close any doors. Perhaps his father's setting boundaries and curbing James' sexual interest had an effect on James' behavior. His behaviors at school were in the middle of the classroom although hidden by a blanket and the children were laughing, thus calling attention to their behavior. This was hardly the behavior of either child molesting the other child or of children hiding secretly to perform forbidden acts.

Generally, children learn very young that behaviors related to sex and sexuality will not be accepted by grown-ups and so don't do them or else learn to hide the behaviors. Neither James nor the other child was ashamed, embarrassed, or denied their behaviors when caught. This was also different than expected. Both boys appeared to think nothing of being caught nor anything about the oral-genital contact.

In a session with both parents, the evaluator shared her impressions gained thus far. While the father was concerned and believed that a change in managing James' behavior was necessary, the evaluator found it difficult to get Jana to agree to any parameters being given to James about his behaviors related to sex or constraints being placed on James' other behaviors. It appeared that her confidence as a parent, while already low, was severely assaulted by the evaluator's suggestions and she became angry and defiant. She didn't want anyone to say anything to James about the sexualized behavior in the classroom or in the bathroom. Neither would she agree to any temporary restrictions on his behavior. She refused the suggestions that either she or the teacher say to both boys, "For a while I would like to make sure you and Peter [the other boy engaged in the behavior at school] stay within sight of the teacher during recess and, please, do not go into the bathroom with each other or other children. It appears you need to remember to not pull your pants down except when you're alone in the bathroom."

During the next session it became clear that James' sexual behavior was still inappropriate when he stood up and said he wanted to go to the bathroom James asked the evaluator, "Do you want to see my penis?" The evaluator hastily said, "No." James reiterated his offer and started to pull down his pants. The evaluator quickly asked him to stop. After taking several deep breaths and hoping that James would resist pulling down his pants, the evaluator asked James if he often showed his penis to people. He seemed undisturbed by the question and said, "Sometimes." When the evaluator inquired further, he said, "My friends." "Any of your friends older than you?" asked the evaluator. "No, grown-ups like you don't seem to want to see my penis," he said without skipping a beat!

This story illustrates how parents who do not teach their children the culturally relevant emotional, physical, and sexual boundaries can confuse the child. Harshness, shame, or guilt regarding engaging in sexual behaviors is harmful to children's growing sexuality; yet, not enough guidance can also be harmful to a child. Children who don't have the same guidance regarding social norms regarding sexuality as their peers will stand out in a manner that makes them unlike the other children in a negative way. It can also make the child at risk for being overidentified as a victim of sexual misuse or abuse.

Another significant risk is that a child molester will see a child with poor physical and sexual boundaries and will suspect previous sexual abuse. Child molesters tend to believe that once a child has been sexually abused he or she is easier to groom for sexual abuse again. You need to provide your children with guidance about the culturally accepted norms of sexual behavior. This will provide a shield for the child and assist them to be compatible with their peers.

CHAPTER 4

Possible Causes of Problematic Sexual Behavior in Children

I believe that virtually all children come into the world with an equal chance to engage in natural and healthy sexual behaviors. There is a wide range of behaviors that can be defined as natural and healthy as there is a wide variation in the behaviors of children due to their inborn differences. Some children have a high sexual interest; other children seem to have almost none, and most are in the middle. Some children feel pleasant sensations in their genitals and some report none. Some children feel sexual arousal as an adult might feel and other children don't. There is a wide range of feelings, interests, and behaviors related to sex and sexuality in children. If we use the definition in chapter 2 to guide us, we will find that most children fit within this definition. Some children don't. Why not? I believe that the main reasons are in the following list.

As children grow up they may develop difficulties with their sexual behaviors. Most problems that occur are due to problems in the child's environment. The following list includes typical environmental conditions that can disrupt the development of natural and healthy sexual behavior.

- Many children are confused based on what they see on television and in movies. It's recommended that you be aware of the shows your children watch and be available to answer questions. Confusing sexual messages are given on television. The messages are often that sex means jealousy, vindictiveness, anger, and extramarital affairs. Values regarding sex and sexuality learned from the soap operas, talk shows, and the movies may lead children to accept abortion as a means of birth control and childbirth outside of marriage as being the norm. These kinds of messages need to be discussed within the family.

- Surfing the Internet can lead children to discover areas of sexuality that they wouldn't find otherwise. Chat rooms discuss sexual issues far beyond the grasp of young children. Invitations to meet and participate in sexual contact have occurred on the Net. Children may even enter adult chat rooms and participate as if they were an adult.

- When left alone children may be with people who expose them to too much adult or adolescent sexuality. Some latchkey kids have a great deal of time to hang out in the neighborhood or with older siblings.

- In some neighborhoods sex is a major influence. When prostitution or drugs are readily available, it's possible that there will be adults with decreased inhibitions who may act out behaviors that are confusing to children.

- Living in a home with a sexualized environment can cause enormous confusion for a child. Some factors that are found in these homes are: parental fights about sex; sexual jealousy of partners; sexual language; sexual jokes; sexual comments about others' bodies; sexual gestures; (negative) sexual comments about men and women; pornography; explicit videos, and R-rated or X-rated movies watched when children are around.

- Some children live in homes where there is little or no physical, sexual, or emotional privacy. For instance: bathroom doors with no locks; children are told the details of their parents' sex lives and problems; children's (over age six) bodies are inspected and discussed, groomed and touched, and they must kiss people they don't like regardless of their discomfort; people don't knock before entering bedrooms or bathrooms; sexual behaviors and nudity occur in living areas of the home regardless of the discomfort of the children.

- In some cases a child's parent is lonely, feels rejected, and turns to their child to meet his or her emotional needs. In cases where the parent's emotional dependency needs are sexualized, the child can feel the parent's neediness and try to respond, or alternately, be frightened and try to get away. Almost like a substitute partner, the child may be brought to sleep in the bed with the parent, hear about the parent's problems, and/or spend time with the parent shopping and/or going to the movies. The parent overexposes the child to his or her own confused sexual attitudes, behaviors, and feelings. This may not constitute overt sexual abuse but covert abuse or emotional incest. It can be highly emotionally, physically, and sexually confusing to the child. The child may feel a generalized sexual tension in relation to the parent.

- Some children live with parents who act in sexual ways after drinking or taking drugs regardless of the presence of children.

- Living in places where sex is routinely paired with aggression, such as in fights about sex, violent sexual language, or forced sex, can be very confusing to children. The effect on children of their parent's behavior is very strong.

- Sexually explicit environments in which sex is used (by the child's parent or guardian) in exchange for drugs or to keep from being hurt sends a message to children. Verbal messages from parents aren't nearly as influential as the messages sent by their behavior.

- Physical abuse and/or emotional or physical neglect is seen in the background of children with problematic sexual behaviors.

- Witnessing physical violence to others, particularly to parents or caregivers and/or siblings in their own home, can contribute to confused sexual thinking and behaviors particularly if sexual language is used.

- Children who have been made to observe others' genitalia or sexual acts for the sexual pleasure of others may be negatively influenced.

- Adults who have observed children or photographed them naked for their own sexual stimulation confuse children regarding sexual boundaries.

- Children who are forced to engage in sex acts together become greatly confused about right and wrong regarding sexual behaviors with other children.

- Children who have been sexually abused by direct physical contact to their bodies may become confused.

- Some adolescents or adults use children to sexually stimulate their bodies. This is an invasion of the child's boundaries and confuses the child regarding his or her rights regarding sexual contact.

When children's emotional and physical space is routinely violated, it may leave an unconscious feeling of distress related to sex, which then manifests itself in increased sexual behaviors. In some children, the level of exposure to adult sexuality has simply overwhelmed their ability to integrate it into their developing sexuality and the children engage in the sexual behaviors to try to diffuse their confusion, tension, and anxiety.

I have given you some food for thought. If your child is engaging in problematic sexual behavior, it will be helpful for you to read the previous list carefully to see if possibly the environment (home, neighborhood, school, church, or day care) in which your child lives has some of these characteristics. If it does you can choose to modify them while assisting your child to modify any problematic sexual behavior.

Remember, if the environment in which your child lives falls on this list, it will be very difficult for your child to change. In some cases it will be impossible. Young children model their behavior after their parents, and the people with whom they live and play. Children with a sexually healthy, loving, and caring home environment rarely "hang out" with sexually unhealthy or violent kids. For more information on modifying problematic sexual behaviors in children, see chapter 7.

Charts on Childhood Sexual Behaviors

The following charts use specific sexual behaviors of children to illustrate how a particular sexual behavior may be *natural* and *healthy* unto itself but when it's characterized by one or more of the twenty characteristics listed in chapter 3, it may be *problematic*. Where the behavior occurs and how it's discovered is also important in assessing the seriousness of a behavior.

These charts are a step in defining behaviors related to sex and sexuality in children of normal intelligence that are *natural* and *healthy*, behaviors that raise concern, and behaviors that require *immediate consultation*. Research by Friedrich (1998) asked mothers about observed sexual behaviors of their children. While not considering as many sexual behaviors nor for the same purpose, with very few exceptions his research provides strong support for these charts.

The charts are not meant for use in the assessment of child sexual abuse. Children engaged in any behavior in any column may or may not have been sexually abused. There are many influences on children's lives that alter their behavior. Not all of them stem from sexual abuse. (See the beginning of this chapter.)

How to Read the Charts

The behaviors in the *first column* are those that are in the expected range. This range is wide—some children may engage in none while some may only do one or two. If a child participates in most or all of the behaviors, this may raise concern.

The *second column* describes behaviors seen in some children who are overly concerned about sexuality, who lack adequate supervision, or live in sexualized environments, and other children who have been, or are currently being, sexually maltreated. When a child shows several of these behaviors, or the behavior persists in spite of interventions, consultation with a professional is advised.

The *third column* describes behaviors often indicative of a child who is experiencing deep confusion in the area of sexuality. This child may or may not have been sexually and emotionally abused or physically maltreated. It may be that the level of sexual confusion and/or aggression in the environment in which the child has lived overwhelmed the child's ability to integrate it. Thus, the child is acting out the confusion. Consultation with a qualified professional who specializes in child sexuality or child sexual abuse should be sought.

Behaviors Related to Sex and Sexuality in Preschool Children

Natural and healthy	Of concern	Seek professional help
Touches/rubs own genitals when diapers are being changed, when going to sleep, when tense, excited, or afraid	Continues to touch/rub genitals in public after being told many times not to do this	Touches/rubs self to the exclusion of normal childhood activities. Hurts own genitals by touching/rubbing
Explores differences between males and females, boys and girls	Continuous questions about genital differences after all questions have been answered	Plays male or female roles in an angry, sad, or aggressive manner. Hates own/other sex
Touches the private parts of familiar adults and children	Touches the private parts of adult not in family, unknown child, or familiar people after being told "no." Asks to be touched himself/herself	Sneakily touches adults. Makes others allow his/her touching, demands that others touch him/her
Takes advantage of opportunity to look at nude people	Stares at nude people even after having seen many people nude	Asks people to take off their clothes. Tries to forcibly undress people
Asks about the genitals, breasts, intercourse, babies	Keeps asking people even after parent has answered all questions at age appropriate level	Asks unfamiliar people after parent has answered all questions. Sexual knowledge too great for age

Erections	Continuous erections	Painful erections
Likes to be nude. May show others his/her genitals	Wants to be nude in public after the parent repeatedly and consistently says "no"	Refuses to put on clothes. Secretly shows self in public after many scoldings
Interested in watching people doing bathroom functions	Interest in watching bathroom functions does not wane in days/weeks	Refuses to leave people alone in bathroom, forces way into bathroom
Interested in having/birthing a baby	Boys interest does not wane after several days/weeks of play about babies	Displays fear or anger about babies, birthing, or intercourse
Uses "dirty" words for bathroom and sexual functions	Continues to use "dirty" words at home after parent says "no"	Uses "dirty" words in public and at home after many scoldings
Interested in own feces	Smears feces on walls or floor more than one time	Repeatedly plays or smears feces after scolding
Plays doctor inspecting others' bodies	Frequently plays doctor after being repeatedly told "no"	Forces child to play doctor, to take off clothes
Puts something in own genitals or rectum one time *for curiosity or exploration*	Puts something in genitals or rectum of self or other after being told "no"	Any coercion, force, pain in putting something in genitals or rectum of self or other child
Plays house, acts out roles of mommy and daddy	Humping other children with clothes on	Simulated or real intercourse without clothes, oral sex

© Copyright 1998 Toni Cavanagh Johnson, Ph.D.

Behaviors Related to Sex and Sexuality in Kindergarten Through Fourth Grade Children

Natural and healthy	Of concern	Seek professional help
Asks about the genitals, breasts, intercourse, babies	Shows fear or anxiety about sexual topics	Endless questions about sex after curiosity satisfied. Sexual knowledge too great for age
Interested in watching/peeking at people doing bathroom functions	Keeps getting caught watching/peeking at others doing bathroom functions	Refuses to leave people alone in bathroom
Uses "dirty" words for bathroom functions, genitals, and sex	Uses "dirty" words with adults after parent consistently says "no," punishes child, and uses healthy language themselves	Continues use of "dirty" words even after exclusion from school and activities
Plays doctor, inspecting others' bodies	Frequently plays doctor and gets caught after being told "no"	Forces child to play doctor, to take off clothes
Boys and girls are interested in having/birthing a baby	Boy keeps making believe he is having a baby after month/s	Child displays fear or anger about babies or intercourse
Show others his/her genitals	Wants to be nude in public after the parent says "no" and punishes child	Refuses to put on clothes. Exposes self in public after many scoldings

Interest in urination and defecation	Plays with feces. Purposely urinates outside of toilet bowl	Repeatedly plays with or smears feces. Purposely urinates on furniture
Touches/rubs own genitals when going to sleep, when tense, excited, or afraid	Continues to touch/rub genitals in public after being told "no." Rubs genitals on furniture or other objects.	Touches/rubs self in public or in private to the exclusion of normal childhood activities. Rubs genitals on people
Plays house, may simulate all roles of mommy and daddy	Humping other children with clothes on. Imitates sexual behavior with dolls/stuffed toy	Humping naked. Intercourse with another child. Forcing sex on other child
Thinks other gender children are "gross" or have "cooties." Chases them	Uses "dirty" language when other children *really* complain	Uses bad language against other child's family. Hurts other gender children
Talks about sex with friends. Talks about having a girl/boy friend	Sex talk gets child in trouble. Romanticizes all relationships	Talks about sex and sexual acts habitually. Repeatedly in trouble with regard to sexual talk
Wants privacy when in bathroom or changing clothes	Becomes very upset when observed changing clothes	Aggressive or fearful in demand for privacy
Likes to hear and tell "dirty" jokes	Keeps getting caught telling "dirty" jokes. Makes sexual sounds, e.g. sighs, moans	Still tells "dirty" jokes even after exclusion from school and activities
Looks at nude pictures	Continuous fascination with nude pictures	Wants to masturbate to nude pictures or display them

Natural and healthy	Of concern	Seek professional help
Plays games with same-aged children related to sex and sexuality	Wants to play games with much younger/older children related to sex and sexuality	Child or children force others to play sexual games
Draws genitals on human figures for artistic expression or because figure is being portrayed in the nude	Draws genitals on some nude figures but not others or on drawings of clothed people. Genitals disproportionate to size of body	Genitals stand out as most prominent feature of drawing. Drawings of intercourse, group sex. Sadism, masochism shown
Explores differences between males and females	Confused about male/female differences after all questions have been answered	Plays male or female roles in a sad, angry, or aggressive manner. Hates own/other sex
Takes advantage of opportunity to look at nude people	Stares/sneaks to stare at nude people even after having seen many people nude	Asks people to take off their clothes. Tries to forcibly undress people
Pretends to be opposite gender	Wants to be opposite gender	Hates being own gender. Hates own genitals
Wants to compare genitals with peer-aged friends	Wants to compare genitals with much older or much younger people	Demands to see the genitals, breasts, buttocks of others

Interest in touching genitals, breasts, buttocks of other same-age child or have child touch his/hers	Continuously wants to touch genitals, breasts, buttocks of other child/ren. Tries to engage in oral, anal, vaginal sex	Manipulates or forces other child to allow touching of genitals, breasts, buttocks. Forced or mutual oral, anal, or vaginal sex
Kisses familiar adults and children. Allows kisses by familiar adults and children	French kissing. Talks in sexualized manner with others. Fearful of hugs and kisses by adults. Gets upset with public displays of affection. Kisses unfamiliar adult or child	Overly familiar with strangers. Talks/acts in a sexualized manner with unknown adults. Physical contact with adult causes excessive agitation to child or adult
Looks at the genitals, buttocks, breasts of others	Touches/stares at the genitals, breasts, buttocks of others. Asks others to touch him/her on these parts	Sneakily or forcibly touches genitals, breasts, buttocks of others. Tries to manipulate others into touching him or her
Erections	Continuous erections	Painful erections
Puts something in own genitals/rectum for the physical sensation, curiosity or exploration	Puts something in own genitals/rectum frequently or when it feels uncomfortable. Puts something in the genitals/rectum of other child	Any coercion or force in putting something in genitals/rectum of other child. Causing harm to own/others genitals/rectum
Interest in breeding behavior of animals	Touching genitals of animals	Sexual behaviors with animals

Getting Help

After reading these charts, you may have decided your child's sexual behaviors are natural and healthy. However, if you're worried, you can call a qualified mental health professional who is familiar with child sexuality or child abuse and ask for an evaluation. Community mental health centers, university counseling centers, pediatricians, and hospitals may have referrals. If you think there may be a medical problem, call your pediatrician. You can also call child protective services or the police for referrals.

CHAPTER 5

Dispelling Fifteen Misconceptions about Child Sexual Abuse and Children's Developing Sexuality

Unfortunately, many adults and children today believe that virtually all sexually abused children will have significant, long-term problems during their lifetime. Sexual abuse is wrong and no child should ever be taken advantage of in this manner, but the research does *not indicate that all children who are abused go on to have severely damaged lives*. The research on the long-term effects of sexual abuse varies between studies. Some of the factors that have been hypothesized to create more negative aftereffects are characteristics of the abuse itself such as:

- The perpetrator being closely related to the victim
- Many incidents of sexual contact that go on for a long time
- The use of force during the abuse
- Sexual acts that include oral, anal, or vaginal penetration

Not all studies find that these characteristics always result in more negative effects for the victim.

Very important in predicting the outcomes for a particular child are charateristics of the child. Some of the characteristics studied are:

- A stressful life prior to abuse
- The child having developmental or psychiatric problems prior to the abuse
- The child having a poor relationship to his or her parents, particularly the mother, prior to the abuse
- The child having poor problem-solving skills after the abuse
- The child having an inadequate support system before or after the abuse

Studies have found that certain family characteristics are frequently found to be important in predicting more negative outcomes for the child victim. Some which have been studied are:

- Family conflict
- Poor family cohesion
- Parent/s who do not support the child after disclosure of the abuse
- The family having limited problem-solving skills

Misconception #1

Children who have been sexually abused are almost certain to have significant long-term aftereffects.

While all sexually abusive acts can have negative effects, the extent of negative effects varies. For instance, one variable is the sexually abusive acts themselves. Often people don't discriminate between sexually abusive events, and think that any sexual event is as damaging as any other event or as if one or two events could have the same aftereffects as years of sexually abusive acts. There may be different aftereffects for different circumstances—such as an infant whose vaginal area is fondled by her mother throughout her first two years of life, a three-year-old child who was touched on her private parts over her clothes three times by a baby-sitter, a six-year-old child who was fondled on the buttocks by a grandfather two times while she was on a swing, a nine-year-old child who watched pornographic movies while his parents engaged in sexual fondling, and a twelve-year-old child who was forced to massage her stepfather's penis from the time she was ten and told she wouldn't be believed if she told. It's important to keep in mind all of the variables when assessing the effects of sexual abuse; the actual sexual acts are only one of them.

Each child is different before the abuse, the circumstances of each child's abuse is different, the family home and support system the child has are different, and so the effects will be different. The important point is to assess each child individually for the impact on him or her. There are no universal effects of sexual abuse.

If you believe there are always serious aftereffects of sexual abuse it can have a negative effect on your child. Some parents are so sure their child will have serious aftereffects that they anticipate them and thus see them when they aren't present.

For example, if a nonabused four-year-old child touches the penis of another child, a parent or teacher might say, "Don't do that," or distract the child. But if the child has been sexually abused, the parent or teacher might think that the child is "attempting to molest" or "getting out of control." Or perhaps a five-year-old who rubs her genitals at nap time will be left alone, but if it were known that she had been sexually abused it might be considered a "sign" of the sexual molest.

A child's sexual behavior is often the same whether he or she has been sexually abused or not. You can use the charts in chapter 4 and the twenty characteristics of sexual behaviors in chapter 3 to determine if there may be a problem with your child's sexual behaviors. If you think there is, you can seek a consultation with someone experienced in working with children who have been sexually abused. If there is no indication of a problem, relax.

The decision in a family law courtroom in 1999 demonstrates the seriousness of this misconception. In a divorce case an attorney successfully argued that because a mother was sexually abused as a child, custody should go to the father. There was no evidence of any misdeeds on the part of the mother. The decision rested solely on her history of sexual abuse as a child.

The likelihood of serious long-term effects for a child who has (1) lived in a loving and stable home, and (2) is sexually abused a few times without any penetration or force by an offender who is not a family member, and (3) whose family responds by being protective, are minimal.

Misconception #2

Sexual abuse is an isolated event that occurs in an otherwise stable home and the negative effects we see for sexually abused children are due to sexual abuse alone.

Studies of sexually abused children frequently find that one form of abuse is accompanied by other forms of abuse. Sexually abused children often live in homes that do not provide a safe and supportive environment for the children (Rind, Tromovitch, and Bauserman 1998). One article reviewed fifty-nine studies of college students and revealed that while the students who had been sexually abused were slightly less well-adjusted than students who hadn't been sexually abused, the poorer adjustment could be better explained by the family environment than the sexual abuse. This is not to say that the sexual abuse was not bad but that the effects of living in a home with alcohol, and/or drug abuse, and/or violence, and/or neglect, and/or divorces, and/or incarcerations, and so on, were also disturbing to the child's development.

Recent research on family violence illustrates that living in a home where the parents are fighting, where there are threats of physical violence, and where actual physical violence occurs can have severe psychological effects on the children. When these are combined with sexual abuse the effects can be even greater. In California, when children are exposed to domestic violence in their homes, it's reportable to child protective services and is considered child abuse.

It is believed that 30–40 percent of children who live in homes where there is spousal abuse have been sexually abused and up to 60 percent have been physically abused. Approximately 80 percent of children directly witness the violence between their parents/caregivers.

Studies that look at the effects of all forms of abuse on children often find that pervasive emotional and/or physical neglect can have some of the most severe and lasting effects on children.

All forms of abuse to children are bad. The more types of abuse, the more potential hurt to the child.

Misconception #3

Children who have sexual behavior problems have been sexually abused.

In the mid '80s when children with sexual behavior problems became a subject of study, an initial question was whether or not a child needed to have been sexually abused to engage in adult-type sexual behaviors with another child. Soon it was recognized that this was *not* necessary. There are many reasons, other than direct, hands-on sexual abuse, which may foster a child to partake in problematic sexual behaviors.

Children need to discover the world for themselves. When children are overexposed to adult and adolescent sexuality, they cannot make sense of all of this information and may act out their confusion in sexual ways. For instance, when children live with parents or caretakers who leave pornography around the house; or allow friends to watch X-rated movies while the children are around; or engage in violent behavior while using harsh sexual language—this can cause great confusion for the child's sexual development and understanding. While technically these aren't sexually abused children according to some legal codes, these types of environment could be labeled sexually abusive.

This is important to bear in mind when evaluating children with sexual behavior problems. If people believe it is only hands-on sexual abuse that causes children to have problematic sexual behaviors they may continue to ask the child who "touched them in ways that were not okay." The child may believe that someone had to do this for them to act in this way and feel pressure to name someone.

Misconception #4

Almost all children who have been sexually abused will engage in problematic sexual behaviors.

There is a misconception that most children who have been sexually abused will participate in problematic sexual behaviors. This is not the case. Across six studies of preschoolers (the children most likely to manifest such symptoms), an average of 35 percent exhibited sexualized behavior. In fact, it is a concern that a sexually abused child's natural interest in sex and sexuality may be curtailed. It is natural and healthy for children to be curious and explore their sexuality.

Misconception #5

Children who engage in sexual behaviors that are not okay for their age are molesting other children.

There is a continuum of sexual behaviors from natural and healthy to disturbed. If your child is engaging in sexual behaviors that are outside the natural and healthy range, he or she will likely fall in one of three groups (see chapter 6). The three groups include children who are (1) sexually-reactive, (2) engage in extensive, mutual sexual behaviors, and (3) molest other children. Only the last group of children are molesting other children; that is, they're using sex in a coercive way to intentionally hurt someone else. By far the largest number of children engaged in problematic sexual behavior are sexually-reactive children. The next largest group includes children engaged in extensive, mutual sexual behaviors and the very smallest group is comprised of children who molest other children. (See chapter 6.)

Misconception #6

All children feel sexually stimulated when being sexually abused and then go on to seek out sexual pleasure.

Children have a hard time describing their physical sensations while they were being sexually abused. Some children describe pleasurable genital sensations, some describe sexual arousal (those closer to puberty), some describe very unpleasant genital sensations, and others describe physiological arousal (tension, anxiety, other unpleasant sensations) not associated with the sexual abuse.

The more pleasant the genital sensations the child experienced while being sexually abused, often the more confusing. Children may think that if it felt good it was their fault, not understanding that their body simply responded to stimulation. This belief is encouraged by the offender making the child feel responsible and bad. This can make it even more difficult for the child to tell.

While there is no empirical data on the types of sensations children have felt while being sexually abused, the study of college students offers a glimpse at how many children felt sexually stimulated when twelve years old and younger. More of the college students who were sexually abused reported sexual stimulation when twelve years old or younger, but there was no statistical difference between the sexually abused and nonsexually abused groups.

According to the research on college students, overall 22% felt "sexually stimulated as an adult might feel" before they were thirteen-years-old when they were engaging in sexual behaviors *alone*. Thirty-two percent of the students who reported being sexually abused felt adult-type sexual feelings, and 20% of those who didn't report being sexually abused felt this type of sexual stimulation. This indicates that more children who were sexually abused felt adult-type sexual stimulation than nonsexually abused children, but the difference wasn't statistically significant.

This means that even though there was a difference, this difference wasn't large enough to be sure it did not just happen by chance. Therefore it doesn't reflect an actual difference between the two groups.

Misconception #7

Most children who have been sexually abused become sexualized and constantly seek sexual arousal.

Some children experience sexual stimulation that is akin to adult sexual feelings prior to puberty, but most do not. Puberty is the time in children's lives when there is great influx of the sexual hormones. The body changes and the secondary sexual characteristics develop, such as the changes in body shape, enlargement of the breasts, the growth of pubic hair, the advent of sperm, an increase in erections, a greater sensitivity in the genital area. Puberty goes on for many years and occurs earlier in girls than in boys. The average age is between nine and fourteen.

Some parents worry that their young children are seeking sexual stimulation when they're engaging in sexual behaviors with other children. This is often a great worry for parents of sexually abused children. Seventeen percent of all students said they felt "sexually stimulated as an adult might feel." For students who reported sexual abuse the percentage was 18 percent and for those who did not report sexaul abuse, the percentage was 16%. These differences were also not statistically significant.

Misconception #8

Once a child has been sexually abused it is very hard to stop them from engaging in problematic sexual behaviors.

In consultation with me, a child protective service's worker described the masturbatory behavior of a young child on her caseload. The child had been masturbating every day for the past year, sometimes for hours, and had caused physical pain to her own genitals from the excessive touching. The child's foster parents were very disgusted with the child because of it. When I inquired about what had been done to help the child stop the behavior the social worker replied, "She is sent to her room and told to stay there until she stops it." As I expressed puzzlement over this approach, the social worker told me, "Well, you know, the child was sexually abused for a long time." In the mind of the social worker this was an explanation sufficient to explain the behavior and to indicate that the behavior would just continue. This is incorrect and unfair to the child. The child's extreme focus on her genitals is not natural and healthy and the child will not know how to discontinue without help. The message the foster parents are giving is "stop yourself" or, perhaps, "your behavior is bad (disgusting, gross, dirty) and we don't want to be with you. If you stop we will like you." The messages will not help the child and may make her feel more out of control, less loved, and more deserted.

Some people mistakenly believe that all children who have been sexually abused are sexualized and therefore will seek sexual stimulation all of the time. They believe that if a child is engaging in *problematic* sexual behavior it is because they are seeking sexual stimulation. They further believe that if a child is seeking sexual stimulation they cannot be stopped. All of these assumptions are incorrect.

- If a child *is* feeling sexually stimulated while engaging in *problematic* sexual behaviors they can and need to be taught the acceptable limits of this behavior.

- If a child *is not* feeling sexually stimulated while they are engaging in *problematic* sexual behaviors, they can and need to be taught the acceptable limits for sexual behavior.

- If a child *is* feeling sexually stimulated while they are engaging in *natural and healthy* sexual behaviors, they can and may need to be taught the acceptable limits of this behavior.

- If a child *is not* feeling sexually stimulated while they are engaging in *natural and healthy* sexual behaviors, they can and may need to be taught the acceptable limits of this behavior.

All behaviors have limits. Sexual behaviors are no different.

In my experience virtually all children can be helped to decrease problematic sexual behaviors. How well and how quickly they succeed in modifying problematic sexual behaviors will depend as much or more on the adults who help them as on them.

Misconception #9

Almost all adult and adolescent sex offenders were sexually abused as children.

Research points out that most adult and adolescent perpetrators of sexual abuse were not sexually victimized as children. According to Hanson and Slater (1991) who reviewed numerous large samples of adult sex offenders, sexual abuse had been experienced by in 20–30 percent of the offenders. Cooper and Haynes (1996) reported the incidence of sexual abuse in adolescents who sexually offend to be approximately 17–47 percent. Thirteen to 40 percent of adolescents who sexually abuse were physically abused as children (Cooper and Haynes 1966). (The range in the numbers is because different studies find different numbers of abuse victims in their samples.)

Misconception #10

Child sexaul abuse victims become adult sexual perpetrators.

It's commonly believed that the reason adult sex offenders offend is because they were sexually abused as children. While this would seem logical and provide an acceptable and intuitively pleasing answer, it's not true. In fact, researchers have tried for the past twenty years to determine the reasons for adults sexually offending. The possible reasons are extrememly varied. There are many similarities in the backgrounds of sex offenders but many more differences. There are also so many different kinds of sex offenders that it's difficult to pin down the reasons for sexually abusive behavior.

While there's an increased risk of later delinquent and adult criminal activity, most child sexual abuse victims don't go on to become offenders of any kind (Widom and Ames 1994). Research on the impact of abuse find substantial groups of victims who appear to have little or no symptomatology (Sirles, Smith, and Kusama 1989;

Kendall-Tackett, Williams, et al. 1993). When the abusive incident is less severe, or the child has good coping skills, or the child has a good relationship with a significant and supportive person, the negative effects are decreased (Widom and Ames 1994).

In the past, unqualified acceptance of the intergenerational hypothesis (of the transmission of abuse) has had many negative consequences. Most adults who were maltreated have been told so many times that they will abuse their children that for some it makes them. Many feel like walking time bombs. In addition, persistent acceptance of this belief has impeded progress in understanding the etiology of abuse and led to misguided judicial and social policy interventions. The time has come for the intergenerational myth to be put aside and for researchers to cease asking, "Do abused children become abusive parents?" and ask instead, "Under what conditions is the transmission of abuse most likely to occur?" (Kaufman and Zigler 1987).

The best estimate of intergenerational transmission appears to be 30 percent plus or minus 5 percent. This suggests that approximately one-quarter to one-third of all individuals who were physically abused, sexually abused, or extremely neglected will subject their children to one of these forms of maltreatment, while the remaining two-thirds to three-quarters will provide adequate care for their children (Kaufman and Zigler 1987).

During the break in a training I was giving for foster parents on children with sexual behavior problems, a woman approached me. Cautiously, she asked, "Did you say that only a very small percentage of sexually abused children would start molesting children during childhood?" I reiterated my belief that less than ½ of 1 percent of child sexual abuse victims would start to molest other children during childhood. The woman burst out crying. She'd been told by the social worker for her two adopted sexually abused children that there was a 90 percent chance that they would start molesting during childhood. For the four years she had had her adopted elementary school boys she'd never left them alone with each other or other children. I asked if the boys knew why they weren't allowed to play alone or with other children. She replied that they did know, and they want to be able to play with other children more. It's hard to imagine the effect of this type of information on a developing child.

In another case, a young adolescent who was in foster care came up to a trainer (who'd mentioned she worked with adolescents who sexually offend) at a conference for foster families and introduced himself as someone "who would be becoming a perpetrator." This young man had been told there was a 90 percent chance he would become an offender because 90 percent of adolescent sex offenders were victims. These are just two examples of why we need to dispel this misconception. Adolescents who were sexually abused as children and whose families have abandoned them need support as they work to develop healthy sexual relationships. Making them fearful of themselves and their sexuality because of something that happened to them over which they had no control is wrong.

While sexual abuse is not found in 50–80% of sex offenders it can be considered a risk factor. One study of 301 adult male felons found that 68% reported *some* form of childhood victimization. Sex offenders reported higher rates of childhood sexual abuse than other offenders—26.3% versus 12.5% (Weeks and Widom 1998).

A great deal of research is being done on the early childhoods of people who engage in abusive and destructive behavior. It has been found that there's frequently a great deal of disadvantage in their lives. There are often many types of abuse, losses, and insecurities. Much of the study is focused on the early relationships between parents and people who go on to sexually offend.

If there isn't a *secure attachment* the child can (but will not necessarily) encounter more difficulties in later life. A secure attachment means that children know that there's someone who cares about them and who will be there if they encounter problems. That person or persons help calm the children when they're either upset, hungry, or hurt. The children have a reliable, consistent environment upon which they build a picture of the world as safe and nurturing. This doesn't mean that the child gets everything he or she wants all of the time, but it does mean that the child doesn't experience fear, hunger, or hurt without a sense of having someone there to help overcome these problems.

The extreme importance for children to have at least one person in their life who they feel cares about them is becoming evident from the research. Children who grow up never feeling respected or cared about by anyone have a hard time developing a positive sense of themselves and of others and developing healthy relationships.

People abused in all types of ways while growing up often cling to the memory of one person who they felt cared about them. This person doesn't have to be a parent but can be an aunt, grandparent, a caregiver in an institution, or even the man down the street who taught the child about cars. The important aspect of the relationship is that the person showed the child respect.

In some cases, the child didn't even know anything about the adult nor the adult about the child, the child simply felt that the person could see that he or she had value. This memory can keep children going and can stop them from seeing the world and everyone in it as hostile. These children can grow up with no intention to hurt others despite how badly hurt they were themselves.

New studies counter stastics frequently cited by media experts and state legislators that claim a 90% recidivism rate for sex offenders. Unfortunately such unsubstantiated claims that "nothing works," reports Margaret A. Alexander, author of the Wisconsin DOC study, fuel the backward trend in public funding for sex offender research and treatment in the last decade.

The Wisconsin study suggests a dramatic decrease in recidivism rates when child molesters are treated. Overall, in an analysis of 10,988 sex offenders from 79 treatment outcome studies, recidivism for child molesters in most categories was less than 11%.

Alexander also found treatment success in the 1980s contrasted sharply with the 1990s. Re-arrests dropped for treated rapists from 22% in the 1980s to 14% in the 1990s; for treated child molesters who target girls from 17% in the 1980s to 11% in the 1990s; for treated incestuous child molesters from 6% to 3%; and the overall rate for treated nonincest child molesters dropped from 18% to 6%. The one exception to the major thrust of her findings was the category of child molesters who target boys. Treated offenders who target boys were re-arrested at a rate of 18% in the 1980s and 23% in the 1990s. Was there any positive treatment effect with this category? By the fifth year the re-arrest rate for untreated offenders in this category—37.5%—was more than double that for similar offenders who had received treatment—14.5% (Alexander 1999).

Misconception #11

Once a sex offender, always a sex offender.

The media and people unfamiliar with the facts often believe that sex offenders will sexually molest forever and that it's almost impossible for them to stop or be stopped. In the popular media sexual offending is presented as being akin to alcoholism in its resistance to change.

In the popular culture, the translation for people who sexually offend is that they can never be around children again. While the data doesn't support this, it's understandable why people are concerned. However, two recent studies of thousands of sex offenders found current treatments to be effective—especially treatment for child molesters.

Misconception #12

Adolescents continue to offend into adulthood.

A recent study of thousands of sex offenders found current treratments to be highly effective—especially treatment for child molesters. Where recidivism was less than 11 percent in most cases (Alexander 1999). In 1998, Hanson Bussiere cited the recidivism rate in a sample of twenty-thousand sex offenders to be 13.4 percent.

Misconception #13

Sexually abused children will soon become children who molest other children.

Parents frequently come to my office with their sexually abused child asking, in very anxious tones, "When will he begin touching other children?" "Is it safe to leave her with other children?" The reason people think this seems to be a combination of misconceptions. All the victims of sexual abuse become sexualized; have very negative aftereffects; and victims become perpetrators.

There are ten of thousands of victims of sexual abuse in the child population at all times; very few become children who molest other children. Because of misinformation parents worry that if their child has been sexually abused, he or she will go on to sexually molest other children. It's estimated that less than ½ of 1 percent of sexually abused children will go on to molest other children during childhood (Johnson 1998).

Misconception #14

All children who sexually molest other children were sexually abused.

Approximately 50–60 percent of children who molest were sexually abused in a hands-on way; a larger percentage were physically and emotionally abused. While the majority of children who molest other children were sexually abused in a hands-on way, these children have also lived in sexualized environments where they developed very confused ideas about sexuality and its connection to hurt, anger, jealousy, and payback. Other problems in their lives often include a disrupted family life that may include drugs, alcohol, divorces, multiple separations, domestic violence, incarcerations, and so on. (See chapter 6.)

Misconception #15

Children who molest other children will inevitably continue to molest into adolescence and adulthood.

A very unfortunate side effect of the misconception that adults cannot stop sexually offending is that the same is true for children. In some states if a child twelve or younger is apprehended and believed to be a child who molests other children, he or she can be put on a child abuse registry or registered as a sex offender. The result of this can be that the child will be considered a sex offender and will never (different states have different lengths of time the child is registered*) be able to get a job working with children or be allowed certain other types of employment either. The child may never be reevaluated to see if he or she has stopped the sexually abusive behaviors. The belief is simply, once a sex offender, always a sex offender. I have seen this happen many times with children as young as seven years old.

Yes, children who molest can stop molesting. They need help from mental health professionals who are trained to provide treatment for these children. They can help these children learn how not to be abusive. If the child lives with his or her parents, the parents will also need to receive therapy. Unfortunately, because many people believe that adult sex offenders can never stop, they also believe this is true of children. Neither is true.

---

* In Illinois a child can be put on the registry for 50 years.

CHAPTER 6

Children with Sexual Behavior Problems

There are some children whose sexual development goes awry. This is generally caused by events in their lives as well as the types of environmental factors described in chapter 4. Children with sexual behavior problems can generally be categorized into three groups. The three groups are *sexually-reactive*, children who engage in *extensive, mutual sexual behaviors*, and children who *molest other children*.

Sexually-Reactive Children

In the natural and healthy course of child development, the developing body and mind of the child interact with the people and the environment in a compatible way that broadens the child's horizons and increases his or her understanding of his or her world. Essential to the natural and healthy development of sexuality in children is that the children are the active agents of their own exploration and discovery.

If sexual experiences are thrust upon children before they're ready, they'll have no way to understand them. Most of the children who fit in the *sexually-reactive* group have been sexually, physically, or emotionally abused, abandoned, or neglected. Those who haven't been abused or neglected (as well as many who've been abused and/or neglected) have lived in sexually overwhelming environments in which the children aren't adequately shielded from adult sexuality (see chapter 4).

Poor boundaries have overwhelmed the child's developing sexuality. These children are confused about sex and sexuality and this confusion manifests in more frequent and more visible sexual behaviors. These sexual behaviors are generally driven by confusion, fear, or anxiety and are frequently precipitated by stimuli in the environment. Many of these sexual behaviors aren't under the behavioral control of the child. In many cases they erupt from the child without conscious awareness.

J. Piaget, a Swiss researcher in child development, introduced the idea of *assimilation* and *accommodation* (1971). These concepts, which were introduced originally to understand children's cognitive development, can help us understand children's sexual development. Piaget believed that as children explore their world they develop cognitive (mental) structures that help organize their experiences so that understanding can take place. As the child has new experiences, these are assimilated into the developing structures or ways of understanding the world. The structures may have to be modified to accommodate new information if it is different than or an expansion of previously acquired information.

However, when children are bombarded by adult sexual behaviors, they cannot assimilate (or absorb) and accommodate (or fit) these experiences into their developing sexuality. Instead these experiences can disrupt the child's developing understanding of sexuality. Unable to assimilate a traumatic or constantly recurring sexual experience, an accommodation (a way of understanding and behaving) may occur that is contrary to healthy development. For instance, after a child has been used for an adult's sexual pleasure, he or she may believe that this is the role children should have toward adults. The child may incorporate into his or her developing understanding of sexual relationships that in order to get attention, making his or her body available to the other person is required.

While Piaget was interested in children's cognitive (mental) development, the concept of assimilation and accommodation can also help in understanding how a child's developing sexual feelings can be transposed prematurely into adult sexual strivings. Generally from infancy on, children engage in pleasurable touching exchanges with the physical world and people. This is healthy sensuality. With the influx of the sex hormones around puberty, this sensuality, the pleasurable feelings that accompany skin contact, gives way to erotic feelings, sexual excitement, and an increased desire for physical and genital contact with others.

When a child's body and genitalia are repeatedly massaged and used for the purposes of adult erotic pleasure, some children's bodies react to the stimulation and they feel sexual arousal and pleasure beyond that usually experienced by children. Some children are unable to assimilate and accommodate these sensations. They cannot understand them and make sense of them because they're premature for the children's age and period of development. The sexual stimulation floods the child's sensory structure and some of the children are then bombarded prematurely with adult-like sexual desires and strivings.

Some of these children become sexually-reactive and seek out other situations to reexperience this sexual stimulation of which they cannot make sense. Others may feel very agitated and anxious when they remember or spontaneously feel these sensations and then act out these feelings on other children. Some of the prematurely aroused children phobically avoid reexperiencing the sexually arousing sensations and avoid further sexual contact. This can last into adulthood.

Sexually-reactive children engage in *solitary sexual behaviors* and *sexual behaviors with other children* and, sometimes, *with adults*. For the most part, this type of sexual behavior is in response to triggers in the environment that are emotionally overly stimulating or reminiscent of previous abuse or feelings that reawaken traumatic or painful memories. A child may respond directly by engaging in sexual behaviors alone or with others. Pleasurable genital feeling or sexual arousal may or may not be present.

Hiding the sexual behaviors or finding friends to engage in the behaviors in private may not be possible for these children as the sexual behavior is generally a way of coping with overwhelming feelings of which they can't make sense. This type of sexual behavior is often not within the conscious control of the child. In some situations children are trying to make sense of something sexual done to them by doing it to someone else. These children don't coerce others into sexual behaviors but *act out their confusion* on them. Many of these children don't understand their own or others' rights to privacy. While there's no intent to hurt others by the sexually-reactive child, receiving sexual behaviors can be confusing for the other child and feel like a violation or abuse.

Some of these children experience post-traumatic stress reactions. These may precipitate the child into recreating sexual trauma with other children or adults. Sometimes the child will try to replicate previously experienced sexuality in an attempt at understanding what happened to them. Sexually-reactive behavior is generally an attempt to decrease anxiety, shame, guilt, or fear the child feels.

The following examples are of sexually-reactive children. You will see that there is a range of problematic sexual behaviors in this category and that some of the children have been sexually abused and some have been overexposed to sexually confusing environments. Sexually-reactive children may engage in sexual behaviors with the problematic characteristics, from the twenty characteristics listed in chapter 3, numbered 2, 3, 4, 5, 6, 7, 8, 9, 10, 11, 12, 14, and 15. A sexually-reactive child might cause emotional or physical pain to himself or herself. It is also possible that a sexually-reactive child might cause emotional discomfort to other children or adults by acting sexual toward them, but this would not be intentional.

Jenna and the Soap Operas

Four-year-old Jenna is a sexually-reactive child. When Jenna's mother brought her in for an evaluation, the child's behavior was unusually sexualized. When Jenna met a man—even a complete stranger—she climbed into his lap, stroked his face, or put her arms around his neck and snuggled up against him. She often tried to stick her tongue into the mouths of people who kissed her, and made sexual sounds. She spent hours sitting on the couch in front of the television, masturbating while humping her stuffed animals.

Jenna was brought in by her mother, an attractive eighteen-year-old named Jackie. Jackie told the child sexual abuse evaluator that she thought her child had been molested. After several interviews there was no evidence of sexual abuse. What emerged, however, was a picture of a home that was sexually overstimulating with virtually no developmentally appropriate activities for a four-year-old.

The little girl and her teenage mother lived in a one-room apartment with Jackie's boyfriend, Bob. There were no children in the complex and Jenna didn't have a single child friend. Every day, the four-year-old and her mother spent hours watching soap operas.

Before Bob returned from work, Jackie and Jenna did their hair and dressed up to "look pretty for Bob." Frequently Jackie let Jenna wear her makeup. At night, Jenna watched cable movies and slept on the sofa bed where Bob and Jackie made love ("only after Jenna is asleep," Jackie told the psychologist).

Like most sexually-reactive children, Jenna was very responsive to treatment. For Jenna, recovery was fast and primarily involved working with her mother. Jackie put up a curtained sleeping corner for Jenna that created a little more privacy for the adults in the evening. She and her daughter enrolled in a "Mommy and Me" class that provided Jackie with knowledge of a four-year-old's needs and practice in interacting appropriately with Jenna. Jenna started attending nursery school and Jackie took a parenting course at the local community center. Trips to the park, zoo, and library took the place of the soap operas. With the overstimulation of sexual content out of her life, and with Jackie gently prompting Jenna not to do the humping and providing her with an alternate activity, Jenna ceased the humping within three weeks.

Tommy and "Uncle" Frank

Tommy is a nine-year-old boy who is sexually-reactive. Tommy was sexually abused by a man he called "Uncle Frank" who lived down the street. Ever since the abuse, he has shown an intense and anxious interest in anything sexual and his teacher reports some behavior and attention problems in the classroom.

He has initiated oral sex and rubbing penises with an eight-year-old cousin on several occasions. If the other child didn't want to do it he just asked someone else. He *did not* try to force the boy or threaten him into silence. Most of the activities Tommy engaged in with his cousin were ones Uncle Frank had done to him or he had seen while watching pornographic videos with his "uncle."

Again, like most sexually-reactive children, Tommy was very responsive to treatment. In Tommy's case, treatment focused on his sexual confusion and victimization. Being in group therapy with other boys who had been molested was especially helpful. Tommy's parents attended a group that occurred at the same time as Tommy's. They learned ways to help Tommy stop the sexual behaviors (see chapter 7) and got answers to their questions regarding sexual abuse. Within a period of a few months Tommy's sexual behaviors decreased to natural and healthy parameters.

The Frazzled Foster Mom

Jan and Harold Roberts had raised four boys who had all finished college and started families. While the freedom to pursue any career she wanted after twenty-seven years of raising children interested Jan, she decided that she wanted to give back to the community by being a foster parent. Although Harold was less enthusiastic he wanted to support Jan and so agreed. Only five years away from retiring, Harold stipulated that they would only take children who would be placed short-term with them while awaiting adoptive placements or who were waiting to be returned home.

With this agreement between them, Jan and Harold went to the closest foster family agency and signed up to be foster parents. Jan told the agency's evaluator that she didn't want any children who'd been sexually abused. Harold said any children would be fine. Months of special classes specifically designed for foster parents to prepare them for their new task completed, they accepted two beautiful children into their home.

Maria was four-and-a-half-years old, and Steven was just over three. As is the case with many foster parents, the Roberts were unprepared, even after extensive training, for their task. While they'd been told about the effects of emotional and physical neglect and verbal abuse on children, they didn't really believe the trainers. "All they really need is love," Jan had told Harold during the training.

Jan knew how to love children and had successfully raised her four boys. It hadn't been easy for Jan—she had been emotionally and physically abused by the father of her oldest son and had left him, with a ten-month-old infant in her arms, in the middle of the night when he was drunk and threatening to kill her if she didn't have sex with him. After she married Harold, though, their life was stable. Harold was a wonderful husband who respected her. Together they had three healthy boys.

Jan's life with Harold was good. She never thought back to her childhood as it held only frightening memories of abandonment, neglect, emotional, physical, and sexual abuse. The demons of her childhood, however, were soon to be stimulated by Maria and Steven.

The first eight weeks went smoothly for Jan and Harold. As first time foster parents frequently do, they ignored the problematic behaviors thinking they would "just go away with love and caring." Unfortunately, Maria was only confused by the new love and caring she was receiving. What Maria really needed were clear and consistent limits set for her, along with the love.

Maria's behavior indicated problems. She always wanted to sit on Harold's lap and had a curious way of snuggling up to him. Her kisses and hugs seemed too physical, but Harold had never had a little girl and thought he was being overly sensitive. When he tucked her in at night she wanted him to get in bed with her, saying she was afraid to be alone. She liked back rubs given by him but never asked Jan for any. He didn't mention this to anyone, but he was sure something was wrong the day she pushed her tongue into his mouth.

Maria's relationship to Jan was very different. It seemed that nothing made Maria happy. Convinced that she was doing something wrong, Jan tried harder to please Maria. Jan made her cookies, played games with her, read her books, and sang her songs. Maria dismissed all of Jan's attempts at establishing a positive relationship. This was Maria's way of expressing her negative feelings toward her biological mother to whom it hadn't been safe to show her negative feelings and who didn't even pay enough attention to her to notice Maria's feelings.

Not until Harold came home was Maria ever calm. Until then she cried intermittently and seemed angry and unsettled going from one activity to the next as if she couldn't stop and attend to anything. She slept little during the night and only sporadically during the day when she would collapse from exhaustion. But it was the rocking behavior that bothered Jan most.

It seemed that every time Jan turned around Maria was rocking on something. The arms of chairs, table legs, stuffed animals, or anything she could roll up and put between her legs or on which she could hunch. Could she be masturbating? Jan was sure this couldn't be, she was too young—children didn't get sexual that young.

Jan didn't like this behavior and started taking away all of Maria's stuffed animals as a punishment, hoping that the behavior would stop. She didn't talk to Harold about it as he was so happy with Maria and she didn't want to bring up any problems. After all she was the one who really wanted to have the foster children.

Steven seemed fine to Jan and Harold, except that he didn't appear to want much to do with them. He didn't fuss or cry, mostly he kept to himself. His eating habits were strange, though. He never wanted to finish what was given him. He insisted on carrying a bag around with him with his leftovers. He would eat them slowly during the day and night.

Maria comforted Steven in a motherly way. In fact, she would get enraged at Jan if she tried to interfere. Only when Maria became exhausted and fell asleep could Jan or Harold attend to Steven's needs. While somewhat apprehensive of them when Maria wasn't there, Steven seemed pleased at the grown-ups' attention and smiled broadly. Steven too had problems sleeping. He frequently had nightmares and would sleepwalk.

Sometimes Jan and Harold would find both children huddled in the living room only partially awake. Or else one of the children was on the floor in the playroom or in the hall. Sometimes they couldn't awake them from their night terror; other times they looked awake but in a mesmerized state.

When she did it the second time, Harold told Jan about Maria putting her tongue in his mouth. He had thought maybe it was just a mistake the first time, but the second time he was pretty sure it was deliberate. He'd just told her to stop sucking on his neck when she came around to the front of his face and went for his mouth with her tongue sticking out.

Jan and Harold had never shared their fears about Maria with one another or talked at any length about Maria's behaviors that seemed sexual. Like many first-time foster parents they kept thinking they weren't really seeing what they were seeing and hoped if they ignored them, the behaviors would just go away. As they discussed the behaviors they became more concerned. Had Maria been sexually abused? Was this why she was engaging in so many sexual behaviors? Who should they tell? What should they do? Jan didn't tell Harold but she knew that she was starting to dislike Maria and pull back from her. While she didn't know why she disliked Maria, she knew that she'd never felt like this about any child before. She couldn't admit it to herself, or to Harold, and certainly not to the social worker from the foster care agency. What would they think of her?

The sexualized behaviors didn't go away but seemed to accelerate as they told Maria to stop them. She was humping everything in sight, all of the time. Jan and Harold started punishing Maria for humping things and sending her to her room. They removed all of the stuffed animals from her room and then everything else she used to hump. Maria would cry for hours and was becoming more defiant and argumentative with Jan. Harold could calm her down by rubbing her back, at which time she would crawl in his lap and fall asleep.

When the social worker from the foster family agency came to visit one day unexpectedly, Maria was in her room completely exhausted after having rocked back and forth on her knees for a long time. For the past several weeks there was nothing in the room with which to have genital contact, she just rocked back and forth seemingly in a trance. When the social worker witnessed this behavior and heard how long it had been going on she grew very concerned and gave Jan a referral for assessment and treatment. To the social worker it seemed almost inevitable that Maria had been sexually abused. It would be important to find out who the perpetrator was and get Maria help to resolve the abuse.

Jan realized her apprehension over having a sexually abused child when the social worker gave her the referral. Although she managed to keep the panic down when speaking with the social worker, she couldn't when Harold came home. She was sure that all of her negative feelings toward Maria were now confirmed. Maria was just like her when she was her age, even down to the sexualized behavior with adult males. Jan had been repeatedly physically abused for any and all things, as well as for her humping behaviors. Harold tried to understand what Jan was saying but couldn't really fathom the depth of her distress and identification with Maria. Harold told Jan that now that she understood the problem she had with Maria, she'd be able to handle it. Harold didn't agree with Jan that Maria should go to another foster home. Yes, they'd said they didn't want any sexually abused children but now that they had her, he thought it was unfair to turn Maria away. Jan needed to get herself together and remember that she wanted to give back to her community and that this was their commitment. Harold didn't understand what Jan was trying to tell him partly because she couldn't articulate it and also because she believed he was right, that she should just get over it.

After many evaluation sessions with both children and both sets of parents, it was determined that Maria was a sexually-reactive child whose behaviors appeared to be reenacting what she had seen her mother doing. According to the limited information available through Maria and corroborated by family members, throughout Maria's young years her mother had prostituted herself.

Men would come at any time of the day or night to the one room where Maria's mother Rochelle lived with her children. The men provided her with drugs, a little money, and sometimes food, in exchange for sex.

Maria took care of Steven and her mother as best she could. Her mother was usually stoned and frequently abusive both physically and verbally to Maria. While less than three years and eight months, Maria kept herself and Steven alive but the toll on her was enormous. She watched her mother have sex and shed affection on the men who supplied her with drugs. There was frequently little or no food.

While doing this Maria feared for her mother, hated her, and was terrified that she would be hurt, as frequently happened. On two occasions her mother had been beaten up by the men and taken away in an ambulance while Maria watched helplessly. Both times Maria had called 911. Both times the children were placed with Rochelle's mother who denied her daughter had serious problems. Eventually protective service workers took the children into their custody.

The protective service workers wanted to remove Maria from the Roberts' home as they said she had molested Steven. The therapist, however, felt that the behavior wasn't molesting behavior but sexually-reactive behavior and that a period of time with treatment should be tried before separating the children. Maria and Steven were very close. It would have been detrimental to both children to be separated.

The assessment that the behavior was not molesting behavior rested on several issues. The myriad of sexual behaviors seemed directly related to Maria's confusion about sexual and physical boundaries and there was no force or coercion used, no attempt to hide the behaviors, and the behaviors appeared generated by anxiety and fear. Maria's sexualized behaviors toward Harold and Steven seemed explained when Rochelle's prostitution in front of Maria was disclosed.

Maria said during one session with the therapist, "Mommy always sucked and licked, the daddys liked it." In another session Maria said perplexed, "Mommy always did the humping stuff, nobody got mad at her." When looking for the precursors to the humping behavior by Maria, it appeared that she engaged in this behavior in response to sexual scenes on television, arguing on the television or between Jan and Harold, and when there was tension in the home.

Other precursors seemed to be when Maria was angry with Jan or sometimes when she looked despondent, lost, or in a reverie. It soon became clear that Maria was *dissociating* (spacing out) under the same conditions that triggered the sexualized behaviors. A great deal of her sexualized behaviors were occurring without Maria being fully conscious of them. This accounted for her "spacey" look and her apparent lack of response to being told to stop.

While it was a concern that Maria had engaged in the humping behavior with Steven it was also clear from Steven that she hadn't threatened him nor forced him into silence. She'd asked him if she could play Mommy with him. He had said "yes" but didn't like it and therefore was yelling at her to get off. The door was open and she didn't try to silence him.

When Harold came into the room she didn't deny the behavior or even think it was wrong. While this type of behavior by a sexually-reactive child can make another child uncomfortable and make some feel victimized, it's not the intention of the sexually-reactive child to molest or hurt the other child.

The treatment process was initially slow due to Jan's problems. Harold finally pushed Jan into talking with the children's therapist about her childhood problems and overidentification with the disturbed parts of Maria. Jan saw a therapist who worked with her and also sometimes with Harold. Maria's therapist worked with Maria, Steven, and the foster parents and consulted regularly with Jan's therapist. Within six weeks all of Maria's sexualized behaviors toward Harold and Steven were gone. The masturbatory behavior took longer to curb due to the struggles that Jan was having, and additionally to the strong feelings both parents had that masturbation is a sin.

Concerned that the masturabatory behavior continued, the Roberts finally acknowledged that they weren't following the therapist's suggestions and instead were punishing Maria when she masturbated. Once they followed the plan devised with Maria to decrease the humping behavior, it diminished only to be seen in times of high stress.

Jana and Harold agreed to try to keep their arguments in the bedroom and wait until after the children were asleep. In addition when one of the circumstances in which Maria usually started humping came up, they would try to change it if possible. If Maria looked as if she were growing tense, sad, angry, or experiencing any unpleasant feelings, they would say, "Let me know if you feel like reading a book, singing songs together, want to talk about your feelings, go ride your bike, or play a game." These were previously agreed upon between Maria and Jan and Harold as things to distract her when she felt like masturbating. Jan and Harold encouraged Maria to understand that although her mother had not been available to help her when she was scared, now there were grown-ups to help her when she was worried. Maria was helped to understand the situations that precipitated her masturbatory behavior. She began to ask to do one of the agreed upon alternative behaviors with Jan or Harold when she began to feel like masturbating. She also learned to leave situations that made her uncomfortable or just to sit by Jan and Harold to feel safe. As Maria and Steven grew into happy children and Jan was able to integrate all of her childhood experiences, the Roberts decided to adopt them.

Jan, Harold, Maria (age sixteen), and Steven (age fourteen) are a happy family today. Maria continues to be anxious sometimes around arguing and explicit sexuality. With an understanding of the source of the anxiety she is able to calm herself. She has a boyfriend who she cares about. She doesn't believe in premarital sexual intercourse and has been very open with him about this. She's comfortable with kissing and light fondling. Maria's relationship to both Jan and Harold is healthy. She has only limited memory of her enormous struggles when she was young with her biological mother and Jan, and with the problematic sexual behaviors. She knows she wants to be a very good mother and still guards her role as older sister to Steven. Steven does very well academically and is a talented flute player. Steven remains quiet and gentle. His attachment to the family is firm and healthy albeit restrained in its outward expression.

Sexually-reactive children need a coordinated educational and behavioral plan to assist them to decrease problematic sexual behavior. Depending on the severity of the problem, the children will also

benefit from individual or group counseling to understand the precipitating reasons for the behavior. If a child has been abused, an
understanding and resolution of the abuse should be sought. In some
cases the sexual behaviors will remit within weeks; in other cases, it
takes longer. Parents need education and support to assist their child
in decreasing the behavior the child engages in as a wau of dealing
with the abuse the child has received.

Children Engaged in Extensive Mutual Sexual Behaviors

Often distrustful, chronically hurt and abandoned by adults, children
who engage in *extensive mutual sexual behaviors* relate best to other
children. In the absence of close, supportive relationships to adults,
the sexual behaviors become a way of making a connection to other
children. They use sex as a way to cope with their feelings of abandonment, hurt, sadness, anxiety, and often despair. These children
don't coerce other children into sexual behaviors but find other simi-
larly lonely children who will participate with them.

Almost all of these children have been sexually, physically, or
emotionally abused or neglected. They look to other children to help
meet their emotional needs and their need for physical contact. The
children move toward peers in a sexual way to feel safe, to find an
anchor in the chaos of their lives. These children are engaged in
extensive mutual sexual behaviors.

These children have a far more pervasive and focused sexual
behavior pattern than sexually-reactive children and they're much
less responsive to treatment. One of the striking differences between
these children and the children in other groups is their affect—or
more precisely, the lack of affect—around sexuality. Children with
extensive mutual sexual behavior don't have the lighthearted sponta-
neity of children involved in natural and healthy sexual behaviors,
the shame and anxiety of sexually-reactive children, or the anger and
aggression typical of children who molest. Instead, they generally display a *blasé, matter-of-fact attitude toward sexual behaviors with other
children.*

They often have no model for a healthy parent-child relationship built on trust and caring. Many of these children have been
repeatedly physically and emotionally abandoned by their parents
and feel little or no connection or comfort with any adult. As their
sexuality was developing they most likely saw and heard far too
much of their parents out-of-control sexuality. Their developing sense

of self and relationships was intruded upon in a sexual manner. Boundaries were diffuse and the children's needs for privacy and consideration were negated or obviated.

Frequently children in this group confuse sex with caring; they believe that someone will care about them if they have sex with them or that someone who has sex with them, cares about them. Due to their young age, many of these children don't associate sex with sexual pleasure or excitement but with a sustaining life force. Some of these children are simply engaging in extensive sexual behaviors without thinking. Many of the behaviors may be almost mechanical in a vain attempt at emotional equilibrium.

Children in this group were previously sexually-reactive children. Children don't go from being natural and healthy to engaging in extensive mutual sexual behaviors. The children first become confused and overwhelmed by the overt sexuality in their lives. Then some of them move to using sex as a coping mechanism against their pain, disillusionment, and despair.

Imagine a child in a wooden boat in the middle of the ocean with the wind roaring and the waves crashing all around him. He doesn't know how he got there or how to get anywhere else. There is no land in sight. He doesn't know which direction to head in and couldn't do anything if he wanted because he has no oars. His boat is filling with water. Frantically he tries to get the water out of the boat but then, exhausted, he half-heartedly attempts to kick it out with his feet.

In despair he resigns himself to sinking. He's totally alone and scared of what will happen when he dies. As his mind is drifting away, he sees something in the distance. He brings himself out of his lethargy and resignation and leans forward. As he does, a wave crashes over his head and his boat seems sure to flounder. He tries to keep it level and afloat a little while longer.

The small spot on the horizon comes closer and he can see that there's another young child in a similar boat. They wave and gesture frantically to each other. With tremendous luck the boats come together and the children get together in one boat. Together they bail the one boat and feel safer, more secure, but still imperiled. Together they at least have some hope, however slim, that they'll live with some comfort, however transient, and that help will come for them both.

These children may be easy prey to adults or adolescents who would take advantage of their sexual confusion and neediness. Without treatment, some of these children may grow up to have multiple partners, engage in prostitution, or confuse their sexual needs for their sexual rights. While a substantial number live in out-of-home care or have been placed and replaced in and out of their own homes, these children can be birth siblings.

In the mutual sibling incest home, the parents are often very sexual in their interactions with each other and with other family members. Many of these parents are having extramarital affairs and aren't available to meet the physical and emotional needs of their children. The sexual, physical, and emotional boundaries in the home are generally loose. The children's world is sexualized and diffuse and lacking caring, boundary-setting adults. Some of these siblings will sexualize their own relationships and become involved in extensive mutually agreed upon sexual behaviors. The children feel comfort in each other in the face of the parental void and chaos of the sexualized home environment.

Some of the children involved in extensive but mutual sexual behaviors move between this group and the children who are molesting or coercing other children into sexual behaviors.

Children who engage in extensive, mutual sexual behaviors have the following problematic characteristics listed in chapter 3: 2, 3, 4, 5, 6, 7, 8, 10, 11, 13, 15, and 19.

Two Children Adrift

John, a ten-year-old, and Jim, an eleven-year-old, are both boys at a residential treatment facility. Before entering the facility, John lived with his mother and stepfather. John's mother had been physically, emotionally, and sexually abused as a child and had given birth to John when she was seventeen and unmarried. She worked hard to keep John and his sister at home and safe but fell prey to men who took advantage of her and her children. She was physically and emotionally abused by John's stepfather who also emotionally and sexually abused John and his sister.

John was also physically abused on a regular basis by his stepfather who frequently accused him of having sexual thoughts about his mother. Child protective services removed John and his sister from their mother and stepfather because the children were engaging in sexual behavior with one another. The social workers were unaware of the emotional, sexual, and physical abuse to the children when they removed them from their home.

John's sister was placed in a separate institution for fear that he would continue to engage in sexual behavior with her. He was very depressed, anxious, and fearful when he entered the residential center. He began to have angry outbursts that resulted in broken furniture and a loss of status on the residential unit. John missed his sister and asked to see her frequently. He was denied. However, he didn't ask about his mother or stepfather. He wasn't actively aggressive toward staff or other children and although superficially compliant, at most times he was distrustful and emotionally disconnected from staff.

Jim was brought to the residential center after being hospitalized for severe depression and suicidal ideation. He alternated between being physically aggressive with his peers, and being totally withdrawn. He'd been abandoned as a young child by his mother and father and lived off and on in foster care for many years. On several occasions Jim was returned to his mother only to be removed due to her drug and alcohol problems.

Jim was emotionally neglected by his mother and often left alone for long periods when his mother went on binges. While in foster care, Jim was sexually abused by an adult male neighbor. Jim didn't tell anyone about this. When he was returned home he missed the neighbor and tried to go to see him. In the last four foster homes Jim had engaged in sexually-reactive behaviors with other foster children. When they were caught, they were punished.

In one of his foster homes, Jim's hands had been tied to the sides of his bed to stop him from masturbating when he was falling asleep at night. One foster parent told the social worker he must have had the devil in him to be doing sexual behaviors at his age. He was only four.

Late one night a residential staff member caught Jim and John in the bathroom with Jim applying Vaseline to his penis while standing behind John. Jim and John were friends as much as any of the children on the unit. Both were emotionally needy and confused. But Jim was a year older than John, much bigger, more aggressive, and was standing in a position to insert his penis in John's rectum. It was for these reasons that it was decided that Jim was an offender and John was the intended victim.

When interviewed, both boys said it was the other one's idea, both said they wanted to do it, both denied being forced, and both said it made them feel better. Jim was not believed and it was felt that John was intimidated into silence. Jim was removed to a sexual offender treatment program.

Both John and Jim are examples of children engaged in extensive but mutual sexual behaviors. Their sexual contact was being used as a coping mechanism for the depression, disconnectedness, and despair they both felt. Jim started out as a sexually-reactive child, but moved into this group as he became more alienated from his family and more despairing about adults. Sex had become an important part of his life. The only close and comforting relationship he had had was with the neighbor who sexually abused him. Confusing sex with caring and love, he sought out John as a source of emotional and physical comfort. Both boys denied any homosexual feelings. Yet when living in a dorm full of boys, they felt temporary relief while engaging in the sexual behaviors.

John had already engaged in a sexual relationship with his sister before he left home, which was characterized by the same dynamics. He and his sister clung to each other in a sexual way to overcome the abandonment feelings in the highly charged sexual environment of their home. Both children had engaged in many problematic sexual behaviors alone and with other children of the sexually-reactive type before seeking each other out.

Either Jim or John could become a child who molests given further alienation from the social situation in which they lived and from their families. Being replaced again in the abusive and sexually chaotic home could also be a factor in the development of molestation behavior. Because most children who molest come from a home where physical violence and sexuality were frequently paired, there's a higher chance that John might molest someone.

Because few children molest other children, it's possible that neither will progress into more disturbed sexuality. When puberty hits with the rush of hormones, the confusion of the sexual urges and a complete lack of role models for positive and mutually satisfying relationships, either boy may engage in erratic and emotionally hurtful or dependent sexual relationships.

Children Who Molest

Many professionals involved with the care and protection of children find it difficult to believe that children twelve years and younger can molest other children. Unfortunately, they do exist. (Johnson 1988; Johnson 1989; Friedrich 1988)

As a group, they have behavior problems at home and at school, few outside interests, and almost no friends. These children lack problem-solving and coping skills and demonstrate little impulse control. Often, they're physically as well as sexually aggressive.

The sexual behaviors of children who molest go far beyond developmentally appropriate childhood exploration or sex play. Like the children who engage in extensive mutual sexual behaviors, their thoughts and actions are often pervaded with sexuality. Typical behaviors of these children may include (but are not limited to) *fondling, oral-genital contact, vaginal* or *anal penetration* of another child with fingers, sticks, and/or other objects. These children's sexual behaviors continue and increase over time and are part of a consistent pattern rather than isolated incidents. Even if their activities are discovered, they don't, and cannot stop without intensive and specialized treatment.

A distinctive aspect of children who molest is their feelings about sex and sexuality. These children often link sexual behavior to feelings of anger (or even rage), loneliness, or fear. The shared decision making and lighthearted curiosity evident in the sexual play of other children is absent. Instead, there's an impulsive and aggressive quality to the behavior.

In one case, four girls held a frightened, fighting, and crying eighteen-month-old child while another child put her mouth on his penis. The other girls (all aged six to eight) each took a turn. The little boy required medical attention as a result injuries to his penis.

While most of the children who molest are less physically violent, coercion is always a factor. Children who molest seek out children who are easy to fool, bribe, or force into sexual activity with them. The victim child does not get to choose what the sexual behaviors will be nor when they will end. Often the victim child is younger and sometimes the age difference is as great as twelve years since some of these children molest infants. On the other hand, some children molest children who are the same age or even older.

In sibling incest with a boy initiator, the victim is typically the favorite child of his parents and may be of either gender. For girls it may be any vulnerable sibling who may have special significance to one of the parents. In other cases, the victim is selected due to special vulnerabilities, including age, intellectual impairment, extreme loneliness, depression, social isolation, or emotional neediness. Children who molest often use social and emotional threats to keep their victims quiet. "I won't play with you ever again if you tell" can be a powerful reason to keep quiet if the child victim already feels lonely, isolated, or even abandoned at home and at school.

The sexual behaviors of children who molest are frequent and pervasive. A growing pattern of sexual behavior problems is evident in their histories. Intense sexual confusion is a hallmark of their thinking and behavior. Sexuality and aggression are closely linked in the thoughts and actions of these children.

Children who molest seldom express any empathy for their victims. Ten-year-old David, for example, repeatedly explained that he had to slap an eight-year-old girl and call her a "bitch," because she wouldn't stop screaming. "I told her to shut up," he said, "but she just wouldn't stop." Even being discovered in the act of molesting another child doesn't necessarily break down this denial of responsibility. In another case, when his foster mother walked into the room where nine-year-old John was sodomizing his five-year-old foster brother, the older boy immediately announced, "I'm not doing anything."

Even the bathroom games sometimes seen in children engaged in sexual play are markedly different from the disturbed toileting behaviors common in children who molest. Some children who molest other children habitually urinate and defecate outside the toilet (on the floor, in their beds, outdoors, and so on). While many children may mildly resist changing their underwear, some children who molest will sometimes wear soiled underpants for more than a week or two and adamantly refuse to change.

Many of the children regularly use excessive amounts of toilet paper (some relate wiping and cleaning themselves to masturbation) and stuff the toilet until it overflows day after day. The children continue these disturbed toileting patterns even if severely punished for their behaviors.

While children who molest are often obsessively focused on toileting and sexual activities, the normal sexual curiosity and delight in their bodies is absent. Instead, they express a great deal of anxiety and confusion about sexuality. Many children who molest say they do the sexual behavior when they feel "jumpy," "funny," "mad," or "bad." Yet, after the sexual behavior, most report they feel "worse."

Most of the children who molest were victims of sexual abuse themselves, although the sexual abuse had generally occurred years before the children began molesting other children. All of the girl perpetrators studied (Johnson 1989)—females represent about 20 percent of child perpetrators—and about 60–70 percent of the boys (Johnson 1988) had been molested. Many children live in home environments marked by sexual stimulation and a lack of boundaries, and almost all of these children have witnessed extreme physical violence between their primary caretakers. Most parents of children in this group also have sexual abuse in their family history, as well as emotional and physical abuse and alcohol and drug problems.

Whereas some of these children plan the molests, others occur spontaneously or explosively. Some of the offensive behavior of these children can be seen in their sexually explosive and vulgar language, taunts, intrusive sneaky touching, and hugging. Because of their size, some of these children sexually nuzzle the breasts of adults with their faces. Some of the physical feelings these children experience are associated with anger, fear, and residual trauma or stress-related sensations rather than sexual feelings.

Sexual arousal is sometimes evident in the behaviors of these children and sometimes not. The closer the children are to puberty, the higher the probability that sexual arousal is involved. Their sexually abusive behavior may have the aim of alleviating negative feelings that overwhelm them. Sometimes the abuse is to retaliate against the victim. There's generally a chaining of feelings, sensations, and environmental cues that bring on the sexual behaviors in these children. It's usually not solely for sexual satisfaction or pleasure.

Children who molest engage in sexual behaviors with the problematic characteristics numbered 1, 2, 3, 4, 5, 6, 7, 8, 9, 10, 11, 12, 14, 15, 16, 17, 18, 19, and 20 from the list of twenty characteristics in chapter 3.

This group of children is at the high risk for continuing and escalating their pattern of sexually hurtful behavior unless they receive specialized treatment specifically targeting their acting out (Johnson 1989). The following case example will illustrate a child (Aaron) who molests other children and the children he selected to abuse. You will see how he entrapped some of the children and scared other children into the sexual behaviors. Aaron uses threats and coercion and is engaging the children against their will. Notice that the effects on the children vary and have a relationship to how healthy they and their families were prior to the abuse occurring and how it was handled after the abuse was discovered.

The School Bully

Aaron, age nine, is a third-grader. At three he was sodomized one time by his father who'd been physically abusive to him throughout the first three years of his life. The sodomy was discovered because Aaron was bleeding quite profusely from his rectum when his mother came home one day. Aaron's father was also physically and emotionally abusive to his mother who was also very aggressive toward the father. Life in the home was very confrontational and combative. Aaron's mother, Sheila, lifted weights and was an exceptional athlete. After discovering the sodomy, she would have stayed in the marriage, but his father disappeared because the police were notified by the hospital when Aaron disclosed the sodomy during the medical exam.

Aaron's mother felt it was an invasion of the privacy of her home when the authorities were brought into the situation. While she felt that Aaron's father was wrong to sodomize their son, she said she could handle the father and that he would never do it again. She blamed the police and social services for destroying her marriage.

Before he started the third grade at the neighborhood school, Aaron had been expelled from four private schools due to his threatening, coercive, and assaultive physical behaviors toward teachers and children, and the sexual behaviors in which he was involved. His sexual behaviors included touching his own genitals and those of other children, exposing his genitals on the playground and in the classroom, and disruptive and assaultive sexual language toward teachers and students. This behavior had been continuous since he was five years old.

His third-grade experience in the neighborhood public school began the day after he was expelled from his fourth private school. Aaron's mother was furious with him. On entering the school, Aaron's mother was forthright with the information that Aaron was a "pain in the neck, had no friends, hit kids, and was expelled for sexual behaviors." The school, however, took no special precautions, didn't speak to the other schools, and did not ask for a transfer of records regarding Aaron.

Four of Aaron's classmates were sexually abused by him, three were physically abused by him. The boys were: José, Ted, Greg, and Nicholas, all ages eight and nine.

José was a young child for his grade. His home life was very disrupted by a physically abusive father who drank too much. José's grades were always a struggle, but he tried very hard. His only friend was Ted with whom he played much of the time. Ted was also sexually abused, by his uncle when he was five. Neither José nor Ted were leaders in the class. They were somewhat isolated from the other children.

Their home life was similar and they lived on the same block. Their mothers were friends. Both mothers were struggling with the abusive men in their lives as well as their own upbringing that was plagued by excessive alcohol, abuse, frustration, low income, and multiple incarcerations of family members. They cared a lot for their children but were consumed by the task of keeping the family together. Daily life was a struggle for both women.

Greg was a fairly good student, had many friends, was a relatively good ball player, and had a cheery and bright disposition. His family was intact although there were many squabbles between his parents. His father had left his mother several times but he always returned. The parents were emotionally abusive toward one another, but when dealing with Greg and his five siblings, were loving.

Nicholas was an average to below average student who excelled in sports. He was bigger than most of the other third-graders and had status in the group due to his prowess in athletics. He was a good-looking boy to whom the third-grade girls were attracted. He was well liked by his teachers who felt he tried hard in his school subjects. Nicholas' parents were consistent in their parenting of Nicholas although their own relationship was somewhat strained at times. All of Nicholas' siblings did well in school.

José, Ted, Greg, and Nicholas were all in the same third-grade class with Aaron. Aaron's problems with assaultive and physically aggressive behavior became evident within several weeks of his entering school. The first incident was when Aaron put his hands around Greg's neck and tried to strangle him. Several children stopped Aaron. Greg had handprints on his neck when he arrived at the nurse's office after the assault.

Aaron punched José several times on the playground, wrestled Ted to the floor in the classroom, and several other of the kids were hurt by Aaron when he pushed them down stairs or hit them with balls on the playground. He grabbed Greg and Nicholas' hair several times and pinched their arms and bottoms. The entire classroom of children was privy to his sexual comments and scatological language.

Aaron's classroom behavior was very disruptive. His teacher had him sit next to her and rewarded any signs of positive behavior, but little progress was made. Aaron's disruptive behavior lasted throughout the school year. He was suspended several times but always came back to his classroom. There was no recommendation for special education services because when he did school work it was adequate.

Aaron had oral-genital contact with each of the four boys twenty-five or more times throughout the school year. These behaviors occurred in the school bathroom, behind the building on the elementary school playground, and on the school bus that they all rode together. Aaron had threatened each of the boys not tell about the sexual behaviors. Some of the threats were that he would kill their mothers, others were that he would hurt them. He also bribed them with very good drawings of Air Force jet fighting planes. The children had told the teacher about the hitting, pinching, and other physical behaviors, but not the sexual touching.

José, Ted, Greg, and Nicholas were supposed to go to summer school but refused. Their parents called the school saying their children were afraid to attend school, but that they didn't know why. After extensive interviews by the school psychologist each of the boys told of the oral-genital contact by Aaron to them. They explained that they were all made to put their mouth on Aaron's penis also. The boys didn't want to do this with Aaron anymore and so refused to go back to school. Each of them was also fearful of the hitting, pinching, and shoving.

Evaluations of the children showed that each of the boys had different reactions to the sexual and physical assaults by Aaron. Emotionally, Ted and José were the most troubled by the behaviors. They were both becoming more fearful, anxious, and distant. It was hard to comfort them and they cried easily. Developmental milestones previously met were lost. Both were having nightmares, wetting their pants in the day, and having frequent nighttime accidents. Ted was getting help from the school counselor. José was seeing a psychologist in the local mental health center. Neither child had told about the sexually abusive behavior.

Greg became more easily intimidated by people and events and was less gregarious. Whereas he'd previously had an interest in everything and showed a voracious appetite for exploring his environment, he was less willing to leave his parents' side. He continued to do well in his daily life at home. Neither Greg nor Nicholas' parents had noticed any behavioral or emotional changes in their sons that concerned them prior to the boys refusing to go to summer school. Nicholas was the least affected and didn't show any behavioral changes.

The Child Sexual Behavior Checklist (CSBCL) (Johnson 1998) was used to assess their sexual behaviors. This list of one hundred fifty sexual and other related behaviors is filled out by the parents or caretakers. As in the emotional realm, the children most effected in the sexual realm were José and Ted. Both children were involved in multiple sexual behaviors. They were touching their own genitals frequently in public and seemed unable to stop.

Their use of sexual language had increased. Ted had tried to touch his mothers' breast, and had been caught pulling back the foreskin of a dog's penis. José had been caught peeking at others in the bathroom and writing a note about sex to a girl at school. Ted and José were both very anxious about sexual topics.

Greg showed some concerning sexual behaviors such as entering the bathroom at home when he knew someone else was using the toilet and showing his privates at home by walking nude in the house. He'd never done this before. He asked innumerable questions about AIDS and other sexually transmitted diseases. He had not tried to engage any other children in sexual behavior. Nicholas' CSBCL showed no sexual behaviors of concern except for a greater than usual amount of sexual talk and jokes.

During the interviews it was disclosed that Ted and José had engaged each other in mutually agreed upon oral-genital contact on four occasions. Also José and Ted had separately asked another child to engage in oral-genital contact. Both had been rebuffed and hadn't pursued it any further. Their anxiety about sexuality was coupled with intense shame and guilt about their sexual behavior with each other. Both children wanted to stop the behavior but described "just doing it." Of the four children only Greg described pleasurable sensations from the sexual behaviors. He said his penis felt "kind of tingly" when he touched it or let it wiggle freely when he walked around. Ted and José said it felt mostly bad when they touched each other.

Generally, the same sexually and physically abusive behaviors occurred to each of the four boys. It's important to see how differently the abuse affected the four boys emotionally, behaviorally, and in regard to their sexual development. The children who were having fewer problems prior to the abuse and whose families had fewer troubles tended to have fewer problems subsequent to the abuse.

Aaron is a child who molests. Ted and José are sexually-reactive children. When questioned, the teacher of the third-grade classroom said that the children most likely to be chided or hurt during that year were Ted and José. Even before Aaron entered the classroom these boys were more likely to be bossed around and teased by the other children. These vulnerable children had the worst emotional aftereffects and were more affected in the realm of sexuality. José and Ted showed the most problematic sexual behaviors, were the most confused about sex, and had begun to repeat the oral-genital behavior performed on them with each other and each had tried to engage another child in sexual behaviors.

Ted and José are examples of children who are on the more troubled end of sexually-reactive children. If they were separated from their families or there were more intense disruption and lack of parental and family support, these children might move into the group characterized by extensive mutual sexual behaviors. They're emotionally needy and neglected children who might try to use sex to cope with their feelings.

Both boys need help to comprehend the sexual and physical abuse by Aaron (group therapy will be helpful for this), to understand sex and sexuality, learn to modify their sexual behaviors, and to become more attached to healthy adults. Their parents need help to work out the family situations and provide for the emotional needs of the children. Sex education will be important. The parents will need guidance to help their children modify their sexual behaviors and assistance in dealing with their feelings related to the abuse to their children. The children need to be taught about their rights and how to access adults when they need help.

Greg is a sexually-reactive child, with future problems than Ted and José. Greg will need help in understanding the abusive behavior toward him by Aaron and prevention work to insure that any further attempts at abuse will be disclosed to adults who can help him. Greg will need sex education and time to have all of his questions answered. His fears about AIDS need to be explored thoroughly. Greg will need to understand his rights and the rights of others related to sex and sexuality as he is confused about appropriate space boundaries and showing his genitals. Greg's parents will need help with their relationship to assure that they're available to him emotionally.

Nicholas' behavior is still within the natural and healthy range. His parents are supportive of him and have handled his more than usual sexual humor by setting limits in it. They encourage him to ask questions about what happened with Aaron. Typical of children who are molested, Nicholas said he didn't tell becasue he thought he would get in trouble. His parents told him they understood that children sometimes think this, but they wanted him to tell them when there is anything he feels may not be right.

All of the parents need help to sort through their feelings about the abuse to their children and why the children did not tell them. They'll need education and support regarding how to modify any problematic sexual behaviors of their children. They need to understand behavioral signs to look out for that may indicate further abuse to their children. They will need to know how to talk to their children about sex and, perhaps, sexual education and values clarification about sex. It will be helpful to stress the love, support, and containment children need from their parents.

Understanding the Differences of the Three Groups

It's important to remember the varying response of children to abuse when evaluating children who have been victimized. Not all children respond the same nor need the same interventions, support, information, nor the same length in treatment. In some cases the parents' treatment and support may be longer than the children's.

Attempting to classify children along a continuum is also important to reduce the possibility of mislabeling. In some cases an attempt is made to determine if the child is involved in sexual play or molestation behavior not understanding that there are two other groups of children.

For example, it would be a large mistake to label Ted or José children who molest even though they did engage other children in sexual behaviors that are far too advanced for their age. While they did engage in oral-genital contact with others, they didn't coerce anyone else into the behaviors or show a pattern of sexual behavior that willfully dismissed others' rights.

If you recognize any of the signs of Aaron's behavior in your child you will want to get help right away. You may be worried about calling for help but it is necessary. Find people who you trust to talk to and let them support you as you get professional help for you and your child. Behavior such as Aaron's is highly unlikely to stop without professional assistance.

CHAPTER 7

Taking Action —
How to Decrease
Problematic Sexual
Behaviors

To decrease problematic sexual behaviors such as those described in the case studies of the sexually-reactive children, children engaged in extensive mutual sexual behaviors, or children who molest, there are numerous steps that you can take. Included in this chapter are lists with specific plans to be aware of, tips on how to develop a plan of action with your child, as well as charts and exercises to help your child with this process. It's helpful to have a therapist or other mental health professional to assist you in this process. If your child is at the far end of the continuum of sexual behaviors, that is, he or she is molesting other children, it will be essential to have a therapist and the local child protective services to assist in helping your child. There is also the possibility that he or she may not be able to remain at home while receiving help if there's danger to other children.

Children whose sexual behaviors are not as worrisome as those described in the case studies of sexually-reactive children, children engaged in extensive mutual sexual behaviors, or children who molest, may not require any help to change. You may need to *redirect* your child for a period of time, and the behavior will cease.

If your child is engaging in behaviors in the second or third column of the charts in chapter 4, the following steps may be helpful. You can read through this chapter and do whatever will be helpful in your situation. If you are working with a therapist you will want to advise the therapist of what you are doing and show the therapist this chapter.

Be cautious so that your child doesn't feel blamed or ashamed about his or her problematic sexual behaviors. He or she should experience any help given as support to change the behavior, not that he or she is bad. If you feel that your child's sexual behavior needs to change, you should discuss this with your child and develop an approach together to change the behavior.

It can be helpful for you to remember something you needed to change about your behavior in the past with someone's help. Then you can give your child the help and support that you needed to change a behavior. Shame and blame never help!

Important Points in Gauging Sexual Behaviors

- *If a child is engaging in worrisome sexual behaviors, a thorough and accurate assessment of the child's sexual behaviors is essential.* Sexuality is fundamental to all individuals and to healthy adult relationships, as well as to the preservation of the species. It's incumbent on all adults to be sensitive to the healthy sexual development of children. If your child's sexual behavior is problematic, assessment is essential.

  Mislabeling a child as a child who molests when the problem is of a lesser degree can have significant reverberations. It may result in the child identifying himself or herself in this way and being put in "sex offender specific" treatment where he or she may be "treated" for sexual offending that did not occur. If the child enters the child protective services system and is placed in out-of-home care with this label, it may cause a child to be removed from home and be placed separately from his or her siblings, and it will be very difficult (if not impossible in many locales) for the child to cast off the label.

  Since some people believe that there's no successful treatment for "sex offenders," it's possible that the child will always be seen as a child (then adolescent, then adult) who molests regardless of years of no offending behavior. The implications for damage to the child are endless. Some states in the U.S. have mandatory sex offender registration for young children.

- *With help, children can overcome their sexual behavior problems.* This includes the parents' caring, consistency, limit setting, and understanding. Children with sexual behavior problems cannot solve the problem themselves. If your child is demonstrating these behaviors, you need to be actively and compassionately engaged in helping him or her. If available, therapy should be sought. The therapist will assist in understanding the conflicts and fears of your child and also provide guidance, support, and information to your family.

  Therapists will work with you and your child as a team in modifying the problematic sexual behaviors. If there's a child protective services worker, he or she will also be instrumental in helping the child. For children, the principal and teacher at your child's school will also be part of the team. If the child is in any type of child care, this person or persons will also be part of the team to help your child.

  While some people believe that a child who has started to act in ways more comparable to adult's sexual behaviors cannot stop, this isn't true. Children need help to curtail problematic sexual behaviors—with help, they *can* do it.

- *Modifying children's problematic sexual behaviors can be quite easy or it may be more complex and take a long time.* Sexual behavior problems in children may be minimal, requiring minor intervention. Other children may be so overwhelmed and confused about sexuality that a more sustained intervention is required. A few children engage in coercive sexual behaviors; interventions with these children will require substantial effort.

  Problematic sexual behaviors are the result of learning and can be unlearned. How long it takes to help your child will depend on many factors such as:
  - How many sexual behaviors are problematic
  - How long your child has been doing them
  - The reasons he or she is engaging in the behaviors
  - How much control he or she has over his or her other behaviors (i.e., the level of impulse control and frustration tolerance)
  - How adults have reacted to his or her sexual behaviors

⋆ Your willingness to be consistent and follow through with helping your child

⋆ The health of the environment in which he or she is living

- *A sexual behavior problem, whether serious or less serious, is only a small part of the child's behavioral repertoire and emotional life.* A sexual behaviors problem must not be allowed to overshadow the whole child, either in the child's self-image or in the perception of the child's caretakers.

- *A child who has very severe sexual behavior problems will generally have other problems that will have to be worked on simultaneously.* Other problems may be: bed-wetting, toilet problems, fears, sleep and eating problems, oppositional behaviors, destructive behaviors, physical aggression, school problems, impulse control problems, poor frustration tolerance, unsatisfying peer relations, poor judgment, intense anger, depression, difficulty trusting others, as well as other problems.

- *Substitute caregivers often have strong reactions to children with significant behavioral problems.* This is natural. Yet it's important to try to remain nonjudgmental and nonpunitive with the children. The time to express the anger, despair, and confusion that may arise in caring for these children is with your spouse, other foster caregivers, in support groups, or with the child's therapist.

- *In many cases problematic sexual behavior is a child's unconscious way to reduce anxiety, tension, or other unpleasant feelings, thoughts, or sensations.* Children with disturbed sexuality may attempt to decrease their uncomfortable feelings by engaging in sexual behaviors. Witnessing fights between their caretakers when foul and angry sexual language is involved, hearing through the walls a parent being thrown against a wall because the parent won't engage in some sexual behavior, repeatedly hearing the sounds of two people having sexual intercourse, watching pornographic movies while the adult caretakers are drunk or on drugs, being aware that relatives are giving sex in exchange for money, attention, food or drugs—all of these create feelings in children. The feelings may be anxiety, shame, fear, guilt, anger, resentment, jealousy, or many others. The pairing of sex with these emotions leaves the child very anxious. When these emotions arise in the child, one way the child may try to decrease the feelings is by engaging in the sexual behaviors.

- *Touching, hugging, and kissing may have special significance for a child with sexual behavior problems.* While all young children need comforting and closeness, it will help to move slowly in these areas to find the comfort zone of the child. Children with sexual behavior problems may initially misinterpret these behaviors. If you feel uncomfortable with the way in which a child is hugging or kissing you, discuss it calmly with the child and teach him or her how to do the behavior so both of you feel comfortable. "I don't feel comfortable with that hug. It's too tight. Let's try again." "I want to give you a hug but it seems you wrap yourself all around me. Let's try a hug where we use our arms and hug around our shoulders." "That kiss feels too much like a grown-up kiss. Let's kiss on the cheek, like this."

  If any of the affectionate behaviors need to be stopped for a while because the child will not take redirection, make sure this isn't for long and that the child is taught how to engage in healthy physical contact as soon as possible.

List Your Child's Sexual Behaviors—Together

- *Make a list of all sexual behaviors of the child.* You should observe your child's behaviors and write down everything he or she does related to sex and sexuality. The list might include such behaviors as masturbating by rubbing up and down on furniture, touching his or her own genitals in public, exposing his or her genitals, peeking in the bathroom while others are using it, or touching the breasts of others (see chapter 2).

  If the child has a mental health worker, a useful tool is the *Child Sexual Behavior Checklist*—Revised (CSBCL) (Johnson 1998). The CSBCL is a list of 150 sexual behaviors of children and twenty problematic characteristics of children's sexual behavior. The mental health worker can administer the checklist to as many people as care for the child. will compare the observations of all parents/caregivers, as well as give their combined view of the child's sexual behaviors. This is a great benefit to treatment planning.

- *Study the sexual behaviors the child does to determine which are problematic.* Chapters 1–4 in this book can help you determine which sexual behaviors are problematic.

- *Prioritize the problematic sexual behaviors that require modification.*

- *Choose one behavior to modify. Do this with the child so that both you and your child are working together.* The first behavior selected should be one that will not be too difficult to detect and stop and that occurs fairly frequently. This way, you and your child can experience success. If your child is engaging in coercive sexual behaviors, these must receive immediate attention. Be clear and specific about the problematic sexual behavior on which you'll be working. If there are multiple caregivers, you should all agree before beginning. Children who agree to changing a behavior and feel part of the decision are much more cooperative and feel much better understood. Most adults can remember when a grown-up wanted them to act differently when they were children and how uncooperative they were when they felt forced, misunderstood, and unjustly accused and punished! (See chapter 2.)

- *With the child, decide how to refer to his or her problematic sexual behaviors.* Some children who simulate intercourse with other children while clothed call it "the rubbing stuff." A child who inserts his or her tongue in someone's mouth while kissing may refer to it as "licking." Create a simple, nonjudgmental, straightforward vocabulary for discussing the behavior with your child. Derogatory terms such as "that disgusting behavior," or "filthy actions," or "dirty play" places a value judgment on the behavior rather than helping to accurately describe the behavior so that it can be decreased while leaving the child's developing sense of self-esteem intact.

- *For a few days make notes on when, where, and with whom the problematic sexual behavior occurs.* You'll see a map in this chapter that can help you and the child figure this out. Note that the term "touching behavior" is used rather than sexual behavior. Frequently children don't think of the behaviors as sexual as they don't have that meaning for them. It's not in the child's best interest to make behaviors sexual if this isn't the meaning the child gives them. "Touching behavior" can be used, if appropriate for the child, to refer to contact behaviors that are problematic and need to be modified. Other behaviors that aren't contact behaviors can be called by their names.

What Starts the Problematic Sexual Behavior?

Children need help in determining the precipitants of their sexualized behavior. You can help your child by observing what happens before he or she feels like engaging in sexual behaviors. Talk with your child to discover the exact precipitants. Your cooperation makes your child feel that you understand how hard this is and his or her need for assistance.

It's very helpful for children to know what brings on their problematic sexual behavior so that they can anticipate the feelings and gain control over their behaviors. If the precipitating situations are ones that your child cannot avoid, then he or she must be aware of them and find ways to control himself or herself when these situations arise, or find ways to alert others of the need for help on these occasions.

Children can feel like acting in a sexual way when they see someone in the bathroom with the door partially open or when they see a woman in a flimsy bathrobe or a man in his shorts. Some children feel like acting in a sexual way when they see pictures of people scantily dressed, watch soap operas, or when they hear music with explicit sexuality or sexual connotations.

Other children want to act in a sexual way when they see aggression in movies, videos, or on television. These children may become very anxious when they anticipate aggression in their presence. Due to the volatile nature of many of the initial caretakers of children with problematic sexual behavior, a simple verbal argument between adult caretakers can frighten a child. They may remember how, in their past, even a small disagreement could erupt into intense physical violence, seemingly without warning. Because of this, the child may attempt to intervene to try to stop "the fight" between parents/caretakers or may act in a sexual or aggressive manner to decrease their own anxiety that something bad is about to happen. (See chapter 2.)

The child may have recollections of people or relationships that precipitate problematic sexual behaviors. These are harder to discover and are usually part of the work of therapy. The attitudes or gestures of a person may summon up in the child uncomfortable memories that the child will try to get rid of by acting in sexual or aggressive ways.

Some children react negatively to persons in certain roles because of their past associations to people in these roles. Some children fear or dislike men and feel apprehensive when they are around. For others it may be "mothers," but not all women.

There are children who hate all authority figures and believe they're all mean and unreasonable. This becomes very complex and requires understanding and working through. It can be helpful for substitute caregivers to recognize that the child may not be reacting negatively to them but to persons they may represent from the child's past.

Some children can directly link feelings such as anger, shame, loneliness, intense sadness, or anxiety with the desire to act in a sexual way. One boy who witnessed his prostitute mother being badly beaten by her pimp and then taken away in an ambulance associated loneliness with sexuality and aggression. He could recall the scene vividly and describe how afraid, lonely, and angry he felt at that time. He would say that when he experienced the same loneliness and sadness he felt like doing something sexual and/or aggressive.

Other children have other feelings that precipitate their behavior. This is similar to the classical conditioning explained by Pavlov. When two things are continually paired (or for traumatic events, multiple similar events are related such as sadness, fear, and loneliness with sex and aggression), experiencing one will elicit the other behavior. Children don't realize these things are related. They can't usually tell us without our help. The associations are largely unconscious. We need to observe their behavior and listen to them when they're having trouble to help them find these connections. (See "Mapping Out My Touching Problem" p. 112.)

Develop a Plan to Reduce the Sexual Behaviors

- *Caregivers and the child should agree on how his or her sexual behaviors will be handled.* Together you and your child should agree on what will be said and done if he or she engages in the targeted problematic sexual behavior. Other problematic sexual behaviors should be ignored, if possible, or handled without special attention. It's best to give special attention to one behavior at a time so that the child can feel some accomplishment.

- *Use verbal reminders and cues to help the child modify the behaviors.* You can cue your child with a wink or a nod, or go to the child and say, "We've agreed that behavior isn't okay for young children," or "When you are grown up, those behaviors will be okay, but not now," or "Not now," or "Please stop." As you become attuned to your child's sexual behavior patterns, you'll be aware when he or she is likely to engage in the problematic sexual behavior and can cue the child before anything occurs. Your child should be helped to be more aware of his or her patterns regarding problematic sexual behaviors in order to gain control over the behavior. Your role is to offer him or her the tools and understanding to control his or her own behavior.

If you are touched on the genitals, you can explain, while removing his or her hand, "We don't do that here," or "Those are my private parts and I don't want you to touch me there." Simple, brief statements in a calm and steady voice help children learn your expectations.

- *Encourage the child to come to you if he or she feels the desire to engage in problematic sexual behaviors.* "If you feel like touching someone where you shouldn't (in a way you shouldn't), please come to me and I'll help you get your mind off of it," or "If you feel like touching private parts, leave what you're doing and come ask me for help." You can reward your child verbally for coming to you. Then help to redirect his or her attention from the sexual behavior. You can help your child to defocus from the desire to act in a sexual way by substituting other behaviors. The substitute behaviors should have the following characteristics:

  1. Things the child likes to do and will find pleasurable. The child should be instrumental in determining what these are.

  2. Activities that expend energy. Good activities might be riding a bicycle, skateboard, or a tricycle; playing basketball, kickball, or handball, etc. Activities involving aggression or body contact with another person should be avoided.

  3. Activities that redirect the child's mind from the sexual focus. Playing video games is good for some children. (The handheld video games are very useful for this purpose.) While this doesn't expend physical energy it does require concentration and therefore will distract the child from the sexual feelings and/or thoughts. Other

possibilities are jacks, crossword puzzles, twenty questions, etc.

4. The activity can be solitary, but it's best if you participate with your child. Doing something with you provides a positive motivator for the child not to engage in the sexual behaviors. The sexual behaviors are often to reduce anxiety. It's far better for the child to learn to use positive relationships and interactions with others to reduce anxiety. If you feel that the child is making up their sexual feelings to spend time with you, determine why your child so desires to be with you that he or she will fabricate sexual feelings. In this case, increase the amount of special time spent with your child to see whether this will decrease the fabrication.

- *When you see the child in a situation that may precipitate a behavior or starting to engage in the problematic behavior, offer alternatives.* Go to your child and calmly say, "This may be a hard time for you, let's go for a walk, (skip rope, play basketball or handball, etc.)" or "Let's do something together now," or "What are some of the things that help you at these times?"

  Imagine you have an overeating problem and your spouse and you have agreed that he or she will help you stop by helping you learn when, where, with whom, and how you're feeling when you overeat. He or she will remind you when you get in situations in which you may overeat or when you're overeating, and he or she will do distracting things with you so you won't overeat. Help the child with problematic sexual behaviors in the way you would have your spouse help you. If you can't imagine having a problem with overeating, imagine you smoke or drink too much or take drugs and need help to stop.

- *Encourage the child to understand the types of things that precipitate the problematic sexual behavior and, in a supportive manner, talk about what he or she can do to make the behavior not occur.* This allows your child to manage his or her own behavior, along with your help. Ways your child can control his or her own behavior: He or she can leave places or situations when he or she may want to do the problematic sexual behavior; ask for help; count to ten; breathe deeply and think of something else; find distractions; engage in energetic physical activities to change his or her body sensations; or use any of the substitute behaviors previously listed. (See "My Jobs This

Week" p. 115–116.)

If this, in conjunction with the other suggestions in this book, don't help the child stop problematic sexual behaviors, then consequences may be needed in addition to positive reinforcement.

- *Consequences may be necessary.* You and your child should decide what consequences will help him or her remember to stop the problematic sexual behavior. The level of severity of the consequence should be in proportion to the seriousness of the sexual behavior. The most serious behaviors are those in which the child bribes, cajoles, or threatens a vulnerable child into the sexual activity. The child should understand the seriousness of the behaviors but not be shamed and condemned.

- *Frequently, the sexual behaviors disappear within several weeks or months of an active, consistent plan but may reappear under stress.* The behaviors may reappear sporadically under stress, confusion or other strong emotions. The reappearance doesn't mean that the child has been completely set back but that he or she will need help once again.

  The stressors that precipitate the sexual behaviors can be understood and your child can be helped to understand them. You can help assure that these stressors are decreased, as much as possible.

- *If a child who molests is in the home with other children, the other children should know.* In a family meeting, the child's problem with coercing others into sexual behaviors should be told to others so that they'll be forewarned and better protected. The behavior shouldn't be described as anything outlandish or in a way to make the child who molests feel badly. This process is not to shame the child but to give the child more incentive not to do the behaviors.

  At no time should children ever feel ashamed of the sexual behavior problems. This doesn't promote healing. Everyone in the family must know so that if the child tries to act sexual with one of them, they will understand the problem and tell the caregivers. You can compare the behavior to when a child in the family is physically aggressive. All family members should know about this so that they can let the caregivers know if the child is bullying or threatening them. This is equivalent to family members knowing about the child's sexual behavior problem. It helps your child to stop because everyone in the home will agree to let you know if the child approached them or is observed engaging in the problematic sexual behavior.

Every precaution must be taken that the child who molests cannot coerce, bribe, or threaten other children into silence. Children who molest other children can be difficult to stop and may not be able to be managed in their homes or in foster care. The child may need to be placed in a residential setting and specialized treatment may be necessary.

For children with lesser sexual behavior problems, the parents or caretakers should determine how to best help the child stop the behaviors. If a child is engaging other children in sexual behaviors, all children must know how to get the child to stop and to immediately tell the adults.

- If restrictions need to be placed on where the child can go while he or she is working on problematic behaviors, these should be agreed on with the child and then modified as the behavior stops (see p. 118).

- *Weekly, the caregivers should have a special time to talk with the child and the therapist, if available, about the child's progress in decreasing the targeted sexual behavior.* Even if the targeted behavior has disappeared don't assume that it's completely gone. Each targeted behavior should remain at the forefront of the plan for several weeks. Slowly, other behaviors can be added. Only after a month or so of the disappearance should it be dropped from the weekly discussion. Make sure the child feels pride in decreasing his or her sexual behavior. Any lapses should be seen as just that—lapses. If you become discouraged, so will your child. You are the emotional cheerleaders for your child. But you still need to be consistent with the use of the charts and all reinforcers.

How to Use the Exercises

The use of charts and reward systems can be helpful. You may wish to use the charts to reinforce your child when the targeted sexual behavior doesn't occur. Stars and stickers are helpful and enjoyed by children. The length of time between giving stickers is determined by how hard it is for your child to stop the behavior and the age of your child. The harder the behavior is to stop and the younger the child, the shorter the intervals between rewards.

Your child may receive a sticker two or three times a day, eight to ten times a day, or twenty to twenty-four times a day. With success, the interval can be increased. You can decide if the stickers are rewarding enough or whether your child needs to receive an additional reward in the evening if he or she has earned 75 percent of the total number of stickers possible during that day. You should decide the percentage, keeping in mind that the purpose of the system is to have your child succeed.

Younger or more impulsive children need to be reinforced more frequently than older children have a greater ability to earn rewards and plan for the future, so they can earn a minimum of so many stickers in a three-day, five-day, or seven-day period to receive another reward. Rewards should be *extra* time with adults, such as an *extra* book at bedtime or *more* time with one of the parents or caregivers, such as a walk around the block, a bicycle ride, a basketball game, or a trip alone with the parent to get an ice cream cone. The purpose is to increase the attachment of the child to the caring, nurturing adult, NOT to spend a lot of money.

The chart is a visual reminder of progress and accomplishment. Children should be given verbal praise when they succeed in decreasing the sexual behaviors. Charts must be used consistently in order to be effective. If a child is in therapy, he or she can take the chart to show to the therapist.

Before you start with the charts, complete "Mapping Out My Touching Problem" with your child. This will provide the information you need to fill in "My Jobs This Week."

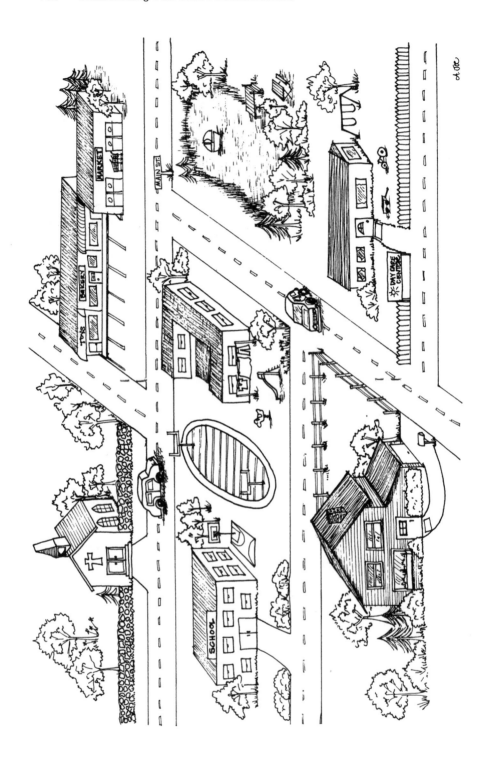

MAPPING OUT MY TOUCHING PROBLEM

SOME OF THE TOUCHING I DO:

_____

_____

_____

_____

I DO THIS TOUCHING ALL ALONE:

_____

_____

_____

I DO THIS KIND OF TOUCHING WITH OTHERS:

_____

_____

_____

THE PEOPLE I DO THE TOUCHING WITH ARE:

_____

_____

_____

_____

I HAVE MARKED ON THE MAP WHERE I DO THE TOUCHING:

_____

_____

_____

THE TOUCHING I THINK I NEED TO CHANGE:

_____

_____

_____

THE TOUCHING PROBLEM I WANT TO WORK ON NOW:

_____

_____

I FEEL LIKE DOING THE PROBLEM TOUCHING

* WHEN I FEEL: _____

* WHEN I AM WITH: _____

* WHEN I SEE: _____

* WHEN I REMEMBER: _____

INSTEAD OF DOING THE PROBLEM TOUCHING I WILL:

_____

_____

_____

MY JOBS THIS WEEK

THE WEEK OF	MON	TUES	WED	THURS	FRI	SAT	SUN
THE WORRISOME BEHAVIOR I AM WORKING ON IS:							
INSTEAD OF DOING THE WORRISOME BEHAVIOR I WILL DO: 1. 2. 3.							
A POSITIVE BEHAVIOR I CAN MAKE EVEN BETTER IS:							
I GET BONUS POINTS FOR:							

My Jobs This Week

The Week of _____	Mon	Tues	Wed	Thurs	Fri	Sat	Sun
The worrisome behavior I am working on is:							
Instead of doing the worrisome behavior I will do: 1. 2. 3.							
A positive behavior I can make even better is:							
I get bonus points for:							

Create an Environment Free of Confusing Sexual Information or Behavior

Avoid the items that may increase sexual feelings or sexual confusion for your child such as the following:

- Printed material with explicit sexual content. Internet access that allows the children to go to Web sites with sexual material and chat rooms.

- Jokes about sex, the use of sexual remarks or innuendoes, or four-letter words.

- Television shows with sexual content. Daytime soap operas can be very energizing. Avoid shows and movies with aggression, violence, and destruction and stories in which there is both sex and aggression. Many videos and dance shows have a very erotic and stimulating quality to them.

- Cable television, unless very closely supervised.

- Provocative clothing—children should dress age-appropriately. Many children want to look more sophisticated and sexual than their age—discourage this. Young girls should wear shorts under skirts.

- Too much explicit sexual behavior. While it's positive for children to see some welcome home hugs or quick kisses between parents and married caregivers, the child may believe the caregivers are going to continue the behaviors through intercourse or possibly engage the child with them in the sexual behaviors.

- Verbally aggressive behaviors or physically aggressive actions. Aggressive behaviors frequently scare children and/or stimulate thoughts of previous frightening events in their lives. Aggressive and sexual behaviors that occur in real life are far more scary to the children than TV pictures and none of them should be allowed.

There are many adjustments and restrictions to your lifestyle that you must remember when you have a child with sexual behavior problems. Adhering to the following suggestions will help curb your child's problematic behaviors.

- Depending on the level and type of sexual behavior problems, children may need to be supervised with other children. A child who molests shouldn't be out of the view of adults in the company of any vulnerable children. Older, younger, and same-age children can be vulnerable. This restriction should last only as long as the child continues to have problems. A gradual lifting of restrictions as treatment goals are met to test the child's progress while still maintaining safety is developmentally appropriate.

- All bathroom activities must be done separately from other children. Respect for privacy should be observed at all times. Even young children shouldn't bathe or toilet together if one of them has problematic sexual behaviors. Locks on the inside of the bathroom doors may be necessary to assure privacy, unless the children are too young to safely unlock the door themselves.

- Walking around nude shouldn't be allowed. Even though this may be normal in children, this should be discouraged by a child with a sexual behavior problem.

- Children shouldn't sleep in the same bed with other children or adults at any time. This can be overstimulating. If there aren't enough beds, a cot or a sleeping bag is preferable. A child who has sleeping problems or problems with bad dreams should be comforted and put back in his or her own bed or in a sleeping bag on the floor in the caregivers' room.

- A child who molests shouldn't sleep in the same room with another child. If this isn't possible, the child shouldn't share a room with another child who is chronologically, developmentally, or emotionally younger, or who is vulnerable to being abused. Motion detectors can be put under the carpet between the beds to help determine if the children get out of their own bed.

- A child may try to molest a child in another room. A buzzer can be used on bedroom doors so that if opened, the caregivers will be alerted. A motion detector can be used that causes the lights to go on or a buzzer or bell to sound.

- Caregivers shouldn't have sexual intercourse when the child is in their presence, even if the child is asleep.

- A child with interpersonal sexual behavior problems should never be left to care for other children, even for a short time.

Encourage Healthy Boundaries

Encourage the development of healthy rules in the home about: the private space that people can have around their bodies when they want it; the private space people like to have for personal things they don't want to share; people's right to privacy in the bathroom, for dressing, and for sleeping alone in bed; private parts; private thoughts; parents' fights being separate from the children; children's right to information about them being shared only with people who need to know; hugs; the use of sexual language; no one being ridiculed because of their body, thoughts, or behavior; people keeping their promises; people not getting out of control when drinking, fighting, gambling, or yelling and about sexual expression.

Encourage the development of healthy physical and emotional contact in the home such as: comforting and soothing touch; touch that takes care of someone's needs; comforting and soothing conversations; communications that take care of someone; or communications that express a need. Examples of healthy touch are: combing, cutting or shampooing someone's hair; shaking hands; high fives; tussling hair; front hugs and sideways hugs; a pat on the back; football; tag; sitting next to someone reading a book; having a young child sit in a grown-up's lap; piggyback; walking hand-in-hand; putting a hand on someone's shoulder; and so on.

Natural and healthy physical contact should be maintained unless a problem arises. Children need to experience positive touch in order to have a healthy development.

Children with sexual behavior problems will benefit by continuous encouragement to respect the boundaries of others and to ask for respect of their boundaries. Children whose boundaries have been violated due to abuse or maltreatment may not recognize healthy boundaries and therefore need to learn them. When their boundaries have been violated children can have a lack of understanding of what they can expect from others regarding their rights to healthy physical, emotional, and sexual boundaries. Children who have been neglected may need encouragement to have emotional and physical contact.

Defining Acceptable and Unacceptable Behaviors for Your Child

It is confusing for a child if sometimes you find their behaviors cute and allow them to happen, but punish the child for the same behavior in another circumstance. All problematic sexual or sexualized behaviors must stop. Children cannot make good decisions about the appropriateness of a time and place, or person.

For an example, a parent may think it's cute or funny when their son is out playing under the sprinkler and trying to pull down the bathing suits of the other children but then punishes the child when he tries to lift girl's skirts on the playground at school. Or the caregivers who think it's cute when a little girl acts in a seductive manner with dad, or mom's boyfriend, but gets mad when she does this with other adults. To the child with sexual behavior problems, these behaviors are similar. It's confusing for them to be alternately allowed and discouraged. Consistency is the key.

CHAPTER 8

Some Areas of Concern to Parents

This chapter lists specific sexual behaviors of children that occur in children with suggestions on how to handle them.

Genital Fondling and Masturbation

In the study of college students it was reported that about 22 percent when six- to ten-year-olds and 31 percent when eleven- to twelve-year-olds stimulate their genitals. This is frequently for the pleasant genital sensations and is often done at bed time. Approximately 22 percent of the college students when eleven- to twelve-year-olds engage in the rhythmic stimulation of their genitals we call masturbation for sexual arousal and pleasure, but only 7 percent when six- to ten-year-olds.

Most parents don't interfere with their children if they confine the touching, fondling, or masturbatory behavior to a place at home away from everyone else. The child's bedroom or bathroom is usually preferable. Some parents find it unacceptable for children to fondle or masturbate. Some parents don't think that it's acceptable behavior for anyone, child or adult. Whatever you believe, you should teach your child. This is your prerogative. The important point to remember is that your son or daughter should not feel badly about himself or herself or get a negative idea about sex or sexual stimulation. If you believe that all sexual exploration should wait until adolescence or adulthood, teach this to your child and explain why you believe this. Open discussion is the key to healthy sexual understanding and development.

Masturbation as a Coping Skill

Children with sexual behavior problems frequently stimulate themselves either with their own hands or by rubbing their genitals on something else or, sometimes, on someone else. This behavior may be for pleasurable sensations, to soothe themselves to sleep, or to reduce anxiety or other unpleasant feelings related to sexual stimuli. Children might also masturbate due to confusion about theirs and others' bodies.

It's natural and expectable for your child to use masturbation in private to either soothe him- or herself, or for the genital sensations. There may be a problem, however, if he or she would rather masturbate than engage in normal play activities. When a child is masturbating to reduce unpleasant emotions or to try to forget their problems, an intervention is probably necessary. Your goal may *not* to stop your child from masturbating completely. The goal is for your child not to masturbate to take care of their worries, problems, fears, and anxieties. If your child uses sexual behaviors in this way this may lead to using his or her body as a way to solve problems when he or she is older. For example, indiscriminate sexual activity, staying in a harmful relationship to have a sex partner, prostitution, alcohol and/or drug abuse, or anorexia or bulimia may be the outcome of this pairing of using the body to decrease tension and anxiety.

How Do I Intervene?

In many cases, the optimal response to anxiety-based masturbation is for you to say, "It seems you're scared (angry, sad, lonely, etc.) and are trying to make the feelings go away by masturbating (

rubbing yourself, pushing on your private parts, etc.). Why don't we read (play a game, make a cake, etc.) instead? There are many things that will make you feel better." Children often don't see people as resources for reducing anxiety or problem solving. You can help your child learn to decrease anxiety by helping him or her figure out what the worries are, and then engaging with your child in fun activities. This is a far better solution for your child than going off alone to masturbate.

If the child is utilizing another person's body for self-stimulation, the simple rule is "It's not okay to rub yourself on other people. Let's go (read a book, play a game, make a cake, etc.)" Some children haven't been properly socialized, while others *may* have been taught to do this for the pleasure of a perpetrator. Teaching appropriate boundaries and sorting through your child's confusion, which leads to the excessive masturbation, will be key to decreasing it.

Compulsive Masturbation

If a child is compulsively masturbating, you should discourage this and provide substitute behaviors (see p. 107) in combination with an active plan to decrease the overall time spent in doing the behavior.

Compulsive masturbation means that the child is preoccupied with masturbation, the behavior is very difficult to interrupt in public or in private, and that it's preferred to more common childhood activities. The child may need to reduce the amount of time he or she privately masturbates in small increments. Periods of time can be allotted for private masturbation, which can then be gradually decreased. If the child is causing irritation to his or her genitals by the masturbatory behavior, a medical consultation should be sought. Or if the behavior seems out of control, a psychiatric evaluation for medication may be advisable.

After problematic masturbatory behavior has been reduced, some children continue to masturbate in private. This may offset sexual behaviors with other children. Masturbation is preferable to involving other children in angry or anxiety-driven sexual behaviors.

Some children completely stop masturbating except when they get scared, highly anxious, or reminded of something that was the initial reason for the masturbatory behavior.

Other children are in the habit of stimulating their genitals and aren't even aware of when they do it. You can discuss this behavior with your child and agree on a cue you will give when he is touching his penis or she is rubbing her vulva. This will help your child become aware of the behavior and stop it. The cue might be a wink or a small nod of your head. This should be a private signal between you and your child and done in a caring and helpful way. Remember to be available to your child to engage in activities or problem-solving to help offset the need for the masturbation.

Same-Gender Sexual Play

Natural and healthy young children participate in sexual play with both genders. The other child is selected because of *mutual interest*, not necessarily gender. For example, if children are going to play "mommies and daddies," they may or may not try to get children of the proper gender. If they want to explore private parts, they may be interested to see if children of the same or other gender look and feel the same as they do.

As children move toward puberty they begin to pay greater attention to the gender of children with whom they engage in sexual behaviors. It's still not uncommon for older children to play sexually with same-gender children and may have nothing to do with choice of sexual partner when the child becomes an adult.

Elementary children may begin to realize that their sexual interests aren't the same as the majority of their friends'. Since most children and adults are attracted to people of the other sex, if a child's interest in sexual contacts is more toward children of the same-gender they may become concerned. Our culture doesn't support same gender sexual contact. This bias against homosexual behavior is generally well known by the time a child is ten, eleven, or twelve years old, and in some families much younger.

If you discover children engaged in sexual behavior, it's important that you react to the *behavior*, not the *gender* of the children involved. It can be very damaging to a child who feels he or she may be gay for a parent to react negatively. Since children engage in sexual behaviors with children of both genders in this prepubertal group, it may have nothing to do with future partner choice. But if it does, negative statements can be detrimental.

Research is leading the scientific community to believe that same-gender partner choice is determined by the genetic makeup of the individual. Although a child can make an emotional choice to participate in postpubertal homosexual behavior, the majority of homosexuality is more likely determined for the individual. In a culture that mostly shuns people who engage in homosexual behavior why would so many people choose to be isolated and put down?

Clothes and Makeup

Raising children in an age where overt sexual expression is all over the television and singers such as Michael Jackson and the Spice Girls appeal to prepubertal children, it's even more important for you to decide on how you want to guide your children's interests—you can discover what they are and encourage them in your child. Otherwise, your child may get caught up in the culture that fosters premature sexualization of children. If there is a void, the media can fill it up.

Foster Healthy Interests

Some children want to collect bugs or rocks, others want to play a musical instrument, while others want to play a sport. When you invest time and energy in any of your children's interests (not your interests for them), you can most likely keep your children's interest in the less desirable cultural icons to a minimum, while developing their interest in something more positive for their own growth.

If you go to your children's school, spend time doing projects with them, or go to their sporting or music events, your children won't need to look for idols from the pop culture to emulate. They'll want to be more like you or your friends who provide realistic models.

Many prepubertal children "fall in love" with pop stars. This may be unavoidable. It's the extent to which a child becomes involved in the pop stars, that is problematic. Children need to develop their own talents and interests and have parents who do that with them. Encourage your children's friendships with children with healthy interests. You can actively (yet subtley) help children to develop make healthy friendships by taking the children on outings together. Making friends with the children's parents and doing group family activities helps also.

Some parents are themselves overly involved in their bodies, makeup, and clothes to the exclusion of a well-balanced life. You need to pay a great deal of attention to the influence of your interests on the development of your children's interests. For instance, if you're very interested in soap operas, your child might begin to act out the roles of the people in the soap operas. Your interests and behaviors are very influential in the development of your children's interests and knowledge. If you read to your children or play games with them at night rather than putting them in front of the television, they'll develop a wider range of interests.

Swearing

Young children like to try out all of the swearwords they hear. Preschool children often say words with absolutely no idea what they mean. If you say to a four- or five-year-old, "You just said shit, what does that mean?" He or she will probably say, "I don't know." Why do they say it? It's fun, funny, and startles adults. This is generally a phase. When they consistently get the message that saying these words isn't acceptable, they say them just to their friends or they stop, for a while. Saying swearwords with their peers isn't going to hurt young people. (See chapter 2.) Using swear words in an aggressive or destructive way is a problem.

When Do I Intervene?

When children say swearwords in front of adults and don't learn to stop, this is of concern. This means that a child is willing to continue to get in trouble for the behavior. There are many reasons for this. You should consider such questions as how consistently are they told to stop? Do people in their own home use this language? Is the child trying to get the attention of someone to say he or she is troubled and needs your help?

Consistency is key—children learn much more directly by words and behavior that are consistent. Therefore, if you say, "Please sit down. Let's read a book, you seem kind of wound up. Is there anything the matter?" You're teaching the child something totally different than the father in the waiting room.

Gender Bending

If children play with the toys usually preferred by the other gender, parents often worry that this is a sign that their child is confused about his or her gender. While this can be the case, it is not valuable to worry or try to change the child. Some parents embarrass, punish, or try to shame the child into changing. None of these tactics are healthy responses to a child who is different than his or her peers.

You can provide a range of toys for your child, and let the child select the ones he or she prefers. Playing with the toys typical to the other gender can be a phase, because of a child's interests or disposition, or simply to bother the parents. Whatever it is, making a big deal of it will only cause a child to become more entrenched in the behavior or feel ashamed about their preferences. Neither will achieve the parents' aim and may cause emotional harm to the child. Generally, when children go to school they conform to their peers—if they don't they get ridiculed. If your child faces ridicule at school make sure he or she understands why. If a child does not want to change the behavior to avoid ridicule, he or she is making a statement. Be open to understanding your child; he or she will then talk to you so that you can help him or her. Don't add to you child's problems. Support his or her individuality.

Girls frequently wear boys' style clothes. This is quite acceptable in American culture. If girls refuse to *ever* wear girls' clothes, this may indicate problems with wanting to be a girl. This can be due to several reasons, such as having been put down for being a girl, or because boys are preferred by the family, because she was sexually abused and doesn't want to appear like a girl because she feels more comfortable in boys' clothes, or because she is making a gender statement. Usually, parents let girls wear boys' style clothes.

However, many parents find it hard to see their son wear girl's clothes. Some boys do like to play dress up with other children and be the mommy. Others like to wear their mother's clothes for fun. Some boys have been forced to dress like girls by parents who didn't want boys. In certain cases boys or girls may feel that they don't want to be boys or girls, although this is very uncommon in young children. Wearing clothes of the other gender is best handled the same as when they want to play with the toys of the other gender—don't make a big deal about it. It is probably advisable to make a deal with your child not to wear girl's clothes outside of the house.

Dating, Parties, and Dances

Communities, families, religions, and cultures have different attitudes about prepubertal children dating and having boyfriends and girlfriends. You have to decide what is acceptable for your family and what the practices are in the child's school, in the neighborhood, and in your faith.

I think that prepubertal children are too young to go out on a date where they are with each other exclusively. Children in the fifth and sixth grades may have after school dances in which groups of children go together to dances and have fun. This is generally considered a healthy way to begin to socialize with the other gender, practice rituals such as going to dances and parties, and talk to peers in a social rather than school setting.

Influence of the Home Environment on Children's Sexual Development

In a home where the parents have moderate attitudes about sex and sexuality and these attitudes are fairly consistent with the majority culture, the influence on the children may be stabilizing. The less consistent the parents' stated (and unstated) sexual values and attitudes are with the majority culture in which the child lives, the more influence the parents may have. However, this influence may not be in the direction the parents want.

This can be true, for instance, when the culture supports dating in adolescence and the parents will not tolerate it. Or, perhaps the school culture allows girls in fourth, fifth, and sixth grade to wear some makeup, but the parents refuse to allow this. Many parents who go against the majority culture find that their children rebel and do what they want when the parents cannot see them. When the parents' sexual behavior and attitudes are such that child protective services or the police would consider them abusive or neglectful, the parents' influence may be at its greatest.

Young children are heavily influenced by their parents' sex and sexuality. So when the parents provide confused messages about sex and sexuality with their own sexual behaviors and practices, this can have a major impact on the development of worrisome sexual behaviors in the child. This influence can start very early and last until someone assists the child to develop sexual attitudes and practices more in concert with the dominant cultural influences, or within the ethnic or religious culture in which the child lives. When the ethnic or religious culture is substantively more restrictive than the majority culture, sometimes the parents aren't able to dominate the child's attitudes beyond about eleven to twelve years of age. As children begin the second period of separation and individuation from their parents and they spend increasing amounts of time with peers, the peer influence can frequently have more influence than the parents'.

How Is Sex Treated in Your Home?

Sex and sexuality is an issue in all homes. Of crucial importance in the sexual socialization of children is the home environment. The manner in which sex and sexuality are expressed and how parents relate to one another varies from family to family. Unspoken messages are often as potent or more potent than spoken messages—actions generally speak louder than words. Parents who go to church and take their children but who also have extramarital affairs and speak falsehoods will likely have a more negative than positive influence on the sexual development of their children.

There is a range of sexual environments in families. They can range from supportive to confusing, or to destructive of healthy and natural sexuality. Think about your own home environment as you read through the following descriptions. How is sex and sexuality treated in your family?

Natural and Healthy Homes

Children are free to express and explore their sexuality, their questions about sex are answered at the level at which they are asked, and the parents are comfortable with their sexuality. Parents touch their children and each other in a loving manner. Family members are respectful of each other's emotional and physical space.

Open or Communal Living Homes

There is an open and free atmosphere regarding sex and sexuality. Sex is good, for the expression of love and caring, and not to be hidden. Nudity may be commonplace. Children are taught about sexual behaviors at an early age and are not discouraged from exploring their bodies and experimenting with others. Parents engage in sexual activities with openness and may share sleeping space with the children. Generally sexual intercourse by adults is done when the children are asleep. Literature about sexuality may be accessible to children.

Sexually Repressed Homes

Sex is not discussed. If a child asks how he or she got into the world, the stork is the answer. Parents don't speak of sex or express their sexuality in front of the children. All sex is highly private—children aren't educated about sexuality even as it regards plants and animals. Any display of sexual behaviors is met with extreme discomfort and highly discouraged. The subject of sex is taboo.

Sex Is Dirty Homes

All questions regarding sexuality are met with hostility. Secrecy around sexuality is forced. Sex is bad, dirty, and never the subject of conversation. Children are made to think they may die or go to hell if they think about sex. Sexual thoughts are the work of the devil. People burn in hell for sex outside of marriage. Sex is only for procreation. Sexual pleasure is sinful. If children are discovered in exploration about sexuality they may be spanked, have their hands restrained from their genitals, or be very closely observed and constantly reminded that sexual play is bad and evil.

Homes with Overt Values and Covert Norms

Sex is positive and to be used to revere God. It's good and healthy to express love in a sexual way with the main goal being to have children. In some cases contraception isn't allowed. Sex outside of marriage is extremely sinful and can lead to being severely punished. Religion is intricately involved in the sexual and social lives of the family members. The overt values and morals expressed are covertly broken by the adult family members. Extramarital affairs are not uncommon and are condoned by the sect members. Abusive relationships are dealt with by the sect members and are hidden from outsiders. Males have the dominant position in the family and religion, women and children are to follow their rules and not question their actions.

In Sexually Overwhelming Homes

There is a good deal of overt sexuality between the parents and their friends. Pornography and other sexually explicit materials may be only minimally hidden, X-rated movies are watched by any family member present, tempers are volatile, men are dominant, women are to do their bidding, and the children aren't adequately shielded from the adults' use of alcohol and drugs.

Sexually and Emotionally Needy Homes

Sex is used as a way to meet the unsatisfied longing of the adults. Generally coming from an abusive and neglectful background, the parents in these families are constantly in search for love, caring, and companionship to fill the void they feel inside. As true love is hard for them to find among the people they attract, sex is the substitute.

Sex is often confused with love and the parents engage in sex to compensate for their emptiness. If a parent is without a partner, a child may be used as a substitute partner. While the parent is usually unaware of using the child as a substitute, the child may feel the pull to fulfill the parent's emotional and sexual needs. Substitution of the child in this role only lasts until an adult is found and then the child is put aside.

Parents using their children as substitutes may have the child sleep in their bed, go out to the movies with them, walk hand-in-hand with them, or invite them to watch television with them. The emotional, physical, and sexual boundaries in these families may be poorly managed.

Aggressive interchanges between the adults are common as the frustration of their needs is not met. One adult may hit the other adult repeatedly. Aggressive interactions between the adults and the children are frequent as the child competes for the attention of the parent and further frustrates the parents' desire to fulfill their own needs.

Sex Is an Exchange Commodity

The parents engage in sex for money, drugs, and other things that they want or need. Children may or may not be used as vehicles for this exchange. Observation of the sexual activities by the children may occur as the parents are not generally focused on the children's needs but on their own. Physical aggression is frequently part of the environment. If the mother is a prostitute, the children may see her beaten by her pimp. Alcohol, drug abuse, and other illegal activities are frequent.

Sexually Abusive Homes

Incest by one or both of the parents occurs. In some cases one of the parents doesn't know that the other is molesting their child. In some cases one parent knows and is unwilling to step in with fervor to stop the abuse. If extended family members live in the home or visit, abuse may be by relatives.

The children who are abused rarely feel they'll get the full support of the nonabusive parent (if there is one) and so endure the abuse. In families where the children do feel they would get the support of the nonabusive parent if they told, the abuser uses threats to keep the child quiet or abuses a young child whose disclosures will be suspect. The abusive parent may use threats of aggression to keep the child quiet. In sexually abusive homes there may be alcohol or drug abuse.

Multigenerational Sexually Abusive Homes

There is concurrent incestuous activity between grandparents, parents, and siblings. Sexual behavior is by the more powerful to the less powerful. While some of the relationships may appear to be mutual, consent is impossible as sexual messages are so pervasive both covertly and overtly that the children are totally confused about sexual expression and its limits and boundaries. Members of the family use physical punishment and physical and emotional bullying as a technique to gain compliance of other family members. The rules for sex and aggression between family members have never been formulated or discussed.

Children whose sexuality is beyond natural and healthy expression may come from any of these families, but very few will come from natural and healthy homes. If they do, it would be due to having been sexually intruded upon by people outside the home.

Sexually-reactive children may have lived in any of the types of homes. Their behavior is a reaction to the overwhelming nature of their exposure to adult and adolescent sexuality.

Children who engage in extensive mutual sexual behaviors have generally lived in sexually overwhelming homes, sexually and emotionally needy homes, homes where sex is an exchange commodity, sexually abusive homes, or multigenerational sexually abusive homes.

Children who molest other children generally come from sexually and emotionally needy homes, homes where sex is an exchange commodity, sexually abusive homes, or multigenerational sexually abusive homes. It is not uncommon that these children were raised in a sexually abusive home for a period of time and then lived with a single parent in a sexually and emotionally needy home.

CHAPTER 9

Sibling Incest —
What Is It?

When siblings (natural, half, step, or adopted) engage in intimate sexual behaviors with one another *over a period of time*, it's called *sibling incest*. Sibling incest can be either forced or mutually agreed upon. Both are very serious and can cause severe emotional problems for the siblings. Sibling incest is not sexually-reactive behavior (see chapter 6) or a couple of sexual behaviors engaged in by siblings. Mutual sibling incest is described in chapter 6 in the section "Children Engaged in Extensive Mutual Sexual Behaviors." Forced sibling incest occurs when one of the siblings is a child who molests and the other child is a sibling victim.

Sibling incest occurs between *brothers* and *sisters*, *brothers* and *brothers*, and *sisters* and *sisters*. More than two children may be involved in sibling incest.

Why Does Sibling Incest Occur?

We do not know what causes sibling incest. There are many reasons that may contribute to the development of this behavior between siblings. If several of the following factors occur simultaneously in a child's life, it can increase the risk of sibling incest occurring:

- Boundaries in the home around privacy and touch are unclear

- Parents are indiscriminate in their selection of sexual partners
- Parents are having ongoing extramarital affairs
- Adults with whom the children live use sex as an emotional crutch
- Exposure to adult sexual behavior which they have not understood
- Other adults close to the family have a significant amount of confusion about their own sexuality
- Parents are emotionally distant
- Parents are not providing a nurturing environment in which the siblings can find love and support
- Exposure to excessive physical aggressive behaviors within the family, including partner abuse
- Exposure to sexually explicit magazines, films, videos, and television
- One or both children were sexually abused
- Siblings were sexually abused together by another person
- Siblings were used in pornography together
- An offender has forced one sibling to be sexual with the other for his or her sexual arousal
- One or both children were physically abused
- One or both children were physically and sexually abused
- Intense rivalry between the siblings that the parents are fostering, sometimes without being aware of it
- Family has always favored the sibling victim
- The sexually aggressive sibling is disliked by the parents
- Sexually aggressive sibling lacks coping skills to deal with feeling angry, anxious, confused, and/or depressd

When two children mutually engage in sexual behaviors many of these issues are important in determining why it happened. It also may be that these children feel "lost" or "abandoned" in their own homes. Children who don't trust their parents or any other adults to take care of them, may look to each other for comfort. This is expressed in sexual as well as other behaviors. This is more likely to happen when there has been sexually confused and disturbed behavior by the adults in the family.

These are some of the reasons siblings may engage in ongoing sexual behavior. The particular reasons for specific children are found by understanding the children, their histories, and the interactional pattern and history of the family. There are always many reasons and many factors involved.

There are homes where many of the previous characteristics may occur but do not encourage or lead to sexual behavior between children—forced or mutual. The factors that come together to foster sibling incest or any other behavior between any two particular children are too complex and multiple to categorize. The personality, temperament, social atmosphere, emotional and economic stressors, interpersonal relationships between all family members, family history, cognitive and emotional strengths and weaknesses, and so on influence all behaviors.

Is Forced Sibling Incest Harmful?

Forced sibling incest refers to a *sibling who is a child who molests.* (See chapter 6.) Sibling incest can have serious short-term and long-term effects on both the child who molested and the sibling victim. When sibling incest occurs, it is crucial that you pay immediate attention to problems within the family.

The sibling victim must be assured that he or she is believed, that he or she will be protected and supported by the parents. It's also important for the child who initiated the molestation to know that his or her behavior was wrong, that there may be legal penalties, and that the parents will work with the child to stop the behavior.

Assistance from professionals outside the family is essential to heal the children and family.

Is Mutually Agreed On Sibling Incest Harmful?

Yes. When siblings become sexually engaged with one another over a sustained period of time it generally means that they're using the sexual behaviors to cope with feelings of loss, fear, and depression. If this behavior continues this can lead to a lifetime of using sex to solve problems. This can lead to promiscuity, prostitution, poor interpersonal and sexual relationships in adolescence and adulthood, depression, anxiety, poor self-concept, eating and sleeping problems. Children engaged in mutual sibling incest are children engaged in sexually-reactive behaviors or in extensive but mutual sexual behaviors. (See chapter 6.)

If the incest behavior appears to be mutual, parents need to firmly state to each child that the sexual behavior must stop and that the parents will get help for the family. The strength of the parents' concern about the incest behavior should be clear to both children.

It isn't always easy to determine whether sibling incest is mutual or forced. This determination will need to be made by a professional. It's not uncommon for one child, usually the younger child, to say that it is mutual due to wanting the approval of the other sibling or being fearful of repercussions. Sibling incest sometimes starts off with one sibling forcing the other and then the victim gets used to the abuse, no longer feels his or her right to say "no," and begins to believe he or she wants it. This is can be especially true if the sexual activity feels pleasurable. The victim child may also like the attention and acceptance from the other child.

How Do Most Parents Feel When They Find Out?

In forced sibling incest, parents' initial feelings are sometimes intense anger at the child who molested, as well as a feeling of betrayal and of having been hurt by their child. Feelings of disappointment, numbness, depression, and confusion often arise. Some parents feel like they'll never love their child again and will never again be able to trust or embrace him or her. A feeling that the child is sick, disgusting, or evil sometimes occurs. Certain parents refuse to believe it's possible. Other parents blame themselves for not paying attention to the signs that this was happening.

When mutual sibling incest is discovered many of these feelings may occur. In some cases a parent may want to designate their preferred child as the victim even if it was mutual behavior. Sometimes the major impulse is to deny that anything happened and believe that a strong rebuke to the children will stop the behavior. This is unrealistic and probably a contributing factor to why the behavior started in the first place.

Many parents find that the discovery of their children's sexual behaviors disrupts their feelings about themselves. Issues from their own childhood that they had buried reemerge and cause them pain and anxiety.

All of these feelings and many more are normal. If you discover that your child has a serious problem it's very difficult. It's important in both mutual and forced sibling incest to find supportive adults with whom to talk. As soon as possible, you should seek therapeutic support for your whole family so the healing process can start. The process of therapy will allow the family members to begin to openly express the multitude of feelings and behaviors that have been hidden.

Don't Deny the Behavior

When sexual molestation occurs between siblings in a family, it's very hard on all the family members. Many parents don't want to believe it happened and instead will deny the reality of the victim and believe the child who molested. As most children who molest deny it, if the parents choose to believe this child, it will leave the child victim feeling alone, betrayed, and confused and the abuse will continue.

Oftentimes parents try to find a conclusion that doesn't force them to face the fact that very serious and emotionally damaging behavior is happening in their family. "Oh, it's just sex play." "Everyone is making a big deal out of this." "I'll punish him or her if it happens again—that will take care of it."

Denial comes in many forms. Parents may try to believe both of the children, the denier and the accuser. In these situations the parents may not do anything and believe it will go away. "It will just go away, if we ignore it." Some parents misguidedly, encourage the sibling victim to change what he or she said happened in order to get the police or protective services out of their family life.

When sexual molestation has occurred between siblings and the initiator of the behavior is not stopped and made to face up to his or her behavior, the behavior will continue. In many cases, the behavior becomes more serious. Receiving no consequences generally strengthens the child's feeling that the sexually abusive behavior isn't really serious and he or she can continue doing it. When the sibling victim is not believed or believed and not protected, serious aftereffects may occur. Effects may include: lack of trust that adults will be protective in the future; a lack of belief in his or her self-worth and right to be protected; depression; anxiety; fear; eating and sleeping problems; drug and alcohol abuse; or other self-injurious behavior.

It is also possible that if either or both parents were victimized when growing up, they may either resolve to protect their children or it can make them apprehensive and uncertain to ask for outside help. People who were repeatedly victimized in their families during childhood and not protected by their parents only need to remember their feelings about themselves and their family members to decide not to let this happen to their children. While asking for help may be hard, the long-term consequences of allowing children to be hurt is greater.

Does This Have to Be Reported?

There is a law that states that all acts of sexual abuse must be reported to the local child welfare agency and/or the police. All professionals who work with children are required by law to report all situations in which they suspect abuse has occurred to a child.

What about Other Children in the Family?

Sibling incest, whether it is forced or mutual, can have a serious effect on other children in the family, particularly if they were aware of the sexual behavior but did not tell their parents. When secrets are kept about serious behaviors, it's an indication of significant problems with the communication channels in the family. It should be determined if there are any other abuse victims in the family. The whole family will have to work on the problem of the incest, trust, safety, and secrecy in the family.

If Incest Happens Again, Will the Children Tell?

One of the goals of therapy for sexual abuse victims is to teach victims prevention skills and encourage them to tell a trusted adult when they need help. Another goal of therapy is to increase good communication in the family. When children believe that there are supportive adults who want to know and who will not blame or punish them, the likelihood of disclosure is greatly increased. This is true even when threats have been used to try to prevent a child from telling.

How Can I Reduce the Risk of Sibling Incest Happening Again?

While each of us influences other people's behavior, we cannot actually control the behavior of another person. The only one who can control a child's sexually aggressive behavior is the child. But if you are the parent, you can do many things to help. The child needs to be very aware that his or her sexual behavior is not *acceptable* and that it *must stop* and that you *will help*. The child should know that therapy is available that will help him or her learn how to stop behaving in sexually inappropriate ways.

You can examine your own part in the genesis of your child's behavior. What are your values, morals, and feelings about sex and sexuality? Are you presenting your children with positive role models in regard to sexuality? How are conflicts solved in your home? Is hurting someone used as a way to resolve problems? Is sex confused with anger, jealousy, or payback?

While the child who molested may want to blame his or her own abusive behavior on the victim, this must not be allowed. However, he or she should also know that while he or she is at fault, there are many things that cause the behavior. The child should know that his or her family will work to make any changes that will help the child reduce the abusive behavior. Helping the sibling victim to gain a positive sense of himself or herself and a sense of his or her own power in relationships in the family will help, if further abuse occurs.

Resources for Therapy

It's very important for the child who initiated the sexual behavior and his or her whole family to be evaluated by a mental health professional who has special training in the field of sexual abuse. In order to locate a professional with training in sexual abuse, call your local mental health facility. Child protective services, the police, and probation departments are other sources of referrals.

CHAPTER 10

Communicating about Sex with Your Child

It's frequently difficult for parents to talk to children about sex. In the survey of mental health and child welfare professionals 33 percent said their parents told them the facts of life when they were twelve years old or younger. Most of these professionals grew up in the 1960s. Surveys of college students growing up in the early 1980s indicate that 43 percent of their parents told them the facts of life when they were twelve or younger. Things are getting better—but not rapidly.

When college students were asked about their primary sources of sex education, 68% said friends, 55% parents, 54% sex education in school, 39% said books, and 34% television. Thirteen percent said sex education came from pornographic material.

Cont. on the next page

When professionals who grew up in the 1970s were asked how much they knew about sexual topics when they were twelve and younger, the average knowledge level was "an incorrect understanding" of the listed topics. They knew most about conception and sexual intercourse. They had almost no knowledge of masturbation, contraception, abortion, and venereal diseases.

When the college students were asked, there was a slightly greater understanding of sexual intercourse, but still in the range on "inaccurate knowledge." The only area in which there was a statistically significant difference between the college students and the mental health professionals was about contraception. Unfortunately, the average knowledge level for both was still in the "inaccurate" range.

Guidelines for Talking with Your Child about Sex

A key to healthy sexuality for your children is knowledge gained from *you*, their parents. You can help your child to sort out their thoughts and feelings and provide them with facts against which to measure all of the information coming to them through their friends, the media, music videos and ad campaigns regarding venereal diseases, and condoms.

When you are comfortable with your values regarding sex and sexuality and openly shares these with your children you're providing an invaluable resource to your child for coping with the pressures of growing up. This is a complex world with many competing sexual mores. The following guidelines can help you in talking to your child about sex. Use those that work for you.

- Children are naturally curious about sex. Their questions should be answered. Listen to the question carefully. You may want to repeat it to make sure you have it right. Answer what they ask. Think about how much they can understand at their age. When they ask a question you may want to ask what they know about it by saying, "What do you think the answer might be?" If this makes a child shy away, answer the question. Sometimes, this approach can clarify misconceptions that he or she may be trying to understand by asking the question.

- Follow the lead of your child. If your child is asking about how animals make babies, talk about that. If they want to understand the entire reproductive cycle, get diagrams and help them understand that. Be sure to stay at the level at which they can understand you. It's probably wise to start with a short answer and then ask if your child wants to know more.

- As children grow up they should gradually learn about sex and sexuality. Be mindful of the age of your children, what they show interest in, and what information they can understand at their age, and then use their natural curiosity to teach them. Be active in teaching your children about sexual topics. When bathing them you can teach the proper names to all body parts. If you're at the zoo and animals are exploring each other's bodies or engaging in sexual activity mention it and explain what's happening. It's easier to teach your children in these more casual ways and your child can absorb information over time. It also teaches your child that you're very available to discuss these topics. This will also make it easier for your child to talk to you if he or she has questions about someone approaching him or her about sex.

- Using accepted terms for body parts (penis, testicles, vagina, breast, uterus, vulva, clitoris, etc.) is recommended particularly with school-age children and adolescents. Start early to identify all parts of the body by proper names, including the genitals. There is no reason to have the incorrect name for any part of the body. You wouldn't give the incorrect name for legs and arms!

- Watch out not to create stereotypes regarding gender roles, such as "Boys are tough," "Boys don't cry," "Boys can take on the important jobs," or "Girls are the weaker sex."

- During the natural course of teaching your children about body parts and functions, differentiate between the penis' function for procreation and urination and the location of the vagina, urethra, and uterus.

- If you decide you want to tell your child the facts of life, make sure you know them and that your facts are correct. If you can't answer some questions, don't make up the answer.

Tell your child you don't know and that you'll find out.
Maybe together you could look up the answer in a book at
home or go to the library.

- Act like a parent. Don't try to be a buddy—your children
  have buddies, they need a parent.

- When you talk about sex or act in a sexual way, be clear
  about what you want to communicate to your child regarding sexual attitudes and values. While children forget a lot of
  things their parents tell them, they generally remember very
  distinctly what their parents say about sexual topics and how
  the parents act sexually.

- If there's any discrepancy between what your own values are,
  how you act sexually, and what you want your child's values
  to be, this can cause your child to be confused, even resentful.
  Be open to discussing the discrepancies, if they exist.

- Stop what you're doing when your child asks you about
  sexuality. If that's not possible, set up a time with your child
  when you will sit down and talk about his or her questions.

- Think about how your parents talked to you or didn't talk to
  you about sex. Is that how you want to be with your children? You can make a choice to be like your parents or to be
  different.

- Many children are reluctant to listen to the facts of life. If
  your child has been sexually abused, he or she may be even
  more reluctant to listen to you. Be sensitive. If your child
  does not want to listen, make sure he or she knows that
  you're willing when he or she is ready. Tell him or her that
  you will try again in a few months. Remember to try again.

- Children are best prepared for responsible sexuality if they
  have positive models and clear values about sex. Children
  pick up most of their values and attitudes by watching the
  adults around them and their peers. Actions speak louder
  than words.

- Find opportunities to bring up the topic of sexuality. For
  instance, if you watch a TV show with your child where a
  sexual issue is raised, ask your child what he or she thinks
  about the issue or state your agreement or disagreement with
  the way in which it's portrayed. The news is full of issues
  about abortion rights, new contraceptives, rape, child molestation, the birth rate in developing countries, women's rights,

HIV, AIDS, etc. If someone you know is pregnant, use this to teach children about the gestation period. If you see animals copulating, explain that this is how animal babies get started. Topics such as sex education in school can be brought up at the dinner table. Be interested in your child's ideas about sex and sexuality.

- Be open-minded. If your values are different than those of your child, discuss this. Parents who refuse to discuss issues, values, and ideals with their children are not valuable resources for guidance and will be disregarded by children. When you engage in a discussion with your child to understand their point of view, and then explain what you believe and why, you can both arrive at a better understanding than either had before. It doesn't compromise values to discuss them.

- Have appropriate books on sexuality available for your children. Read these books together. If your child doesn't want to read with you, assure him or her that you would be happy to discuss any of the topics.

- If your child isn't asking questions about sex and sexuality, make sure you aren't subtly discouraging communication in this area.

- Bring up sexual topics yourself. "When I was young, kids used to talk about sexual things to each other. Is it still the same?" "What do you think about the language in the song, _____?" "Last night on the news there was another bombing of an abortion clinic, what do you think of that?" "Are there any questions you or your friends have about sex I can answer for you?"

- Be aware of your facial expressions and body posture when talking about sex. Children are very sensitive to these cues.

- If you're uncomfortable talking about sex or have negative feelings about sex, get some help for yourself. One of the greatest gifts parents can give children is a healthy attitude about sex and sexuality.

- If you cannot discuss sexual issues with your child but you know someone you trust, you can tell your child that this person is available to talk with him or her about sexuality.

- Remember, children will learn about sex and sexuality. If you don't provide the information, they'll get it somewhere.

While sex education in school is helpful, it's mostly about the "plumbing" and children are generally reluctant to ask questions. Morals and values about sex should come from the family.

- It's important for children to know about the physical changes that come with puberty before they experience them.

- Children need to know about sexual intercourse, reproduction, and contraception before they become sexually active. Tell them your attitudes and values about these matters.

- A way to open up communication about sex with children is to ask what dirty jokes are going around their school. Another technique is to ask about the current sexual slang. This will give you an opportunity to clarify the accurate meaning of slang and the jokes, if your child is confused.

- If your child uses swearwords, you may want to ask him or her what the words mean. If your child doesn't know, you may want to explain the true meaning of slang words.

- It's up to the parent whether or not a child is allowed to swear in their presence. If you swear *liberally* in front of your child, you must be aware that your children will copy you. Punishing your child for what you're teaching them by your behavior is confusing. If you use physical punishment on your child when you're *angry* with him or her, it's useless to tell them not to hit someone else in *anger*.

What to Say When You Find Your Child Engaged in Sexual Behavior

When you're faced with your child engaging in a sexual behavior alone or with another child, you must decide how you want to respond. Do you want to scare your child into never doing it again? Do you want your child to feel he or she has done something terrible? Do you want to distract your child from the behavior and say nothing? Do you want to take the opportunity to teach your child something about touching? Do you want to teach your child the rules you want your child to follow about touching genitals? This is the first decision you must make. When you decide this, what you say and the way you say it will follow naturally.

What Messages Do You Want to Communicate?

What is the *basic message regarding sex* you want to give to two same-age friends the first time you catch them touching each other's genitals in a private, noncoercive way? Which one of these messages would you want to convey:

- Children are curious about sex. It's normal and what you are doing is an example (message 1).

- Children are curious about sex and what you are doing is an example. But I don't think children should touch each other (message 2).

What is the *specific message* you would want to get across to your child right then when you discover children engaged in sexual behaviors?

- Let's take care of your curiosity in another way.
- Stop it, right now!

Positive responses derived from the basic message regarding sex, and the specific message required at the moment, can be one or more of the following. The messages in parentheses address message 2. Where there is only one response it will suffice for both messages.

- "It's okay to be curious (but ask questions, don't touch others)."

- "Children sometimes like to explore each other's bodies (but I don't want you to)."

- "You are getting very interested in your bodies (but keep your interest to your own body)."

- "It's time to go out to play."

- "It's time to go out to play. Are you both okay? (Please don't do that anymore. If you have questions, ask me.)"

- "Is your curiosity satisfied?" stated in addition to inviting the children to do an activity with the parent such as play a game.

- "Do you have any questions you want to ask about bodies?" stated while suggesting they come into the living room.

- "There are lots of ways to learn about bodies, one is by touching someone else, another is by looking in books. If you would like I will show you some books," said while inviting the children to come with the parent to the living room.

Suppose you were to walk in on two same-age children who are good friends who are touching each other's genitals in a private, non-coercive way. This time think of some less positive responses. The following chart provides some examples.

If you say:	The basic message transmitted is:
(Yelling angrily) "Get out of here now. Stay in your room until I can calm down enough to talk to you."	The behavior is really terrible and you're in deep trouble.
"You said you wouldn't do that. I can't trust you ever again."	You are so bad and what you're doing is so bad. I will never believe you again.
"That's disgusting."	Sexual behavior is dirty and disgusting.
"You will be punished for this."	Sexual exploration is bad.
"If I ever catch you again, I'll whoop your ass."	There is something really bad about sexual touching and you deserve to be physically punished.
"Stop doing the nasty."	Sexual behavior is dirty or bad.
"You act like a slut."	Sexual touching is bad and you're really bad if you do it.

Messages in Action

For example, Tim, a father of a nine-year-old boy, finds *Playboy* magazine under his child's bed. What is the *basic message* regarding sex that Tim wants to give his son? "*Playboy* is for adults not children." What is the *specific message* Tim wants to get across to his son right then? "I don't want you to look at it."

Positive responses based on a basic message regarding sex might be: "This is my magazine. These types of magazines are for adults not children, but I guess you found it and really wanted to look. Do you have any questions? I will not leave *Playboy* around. When you grow up, you can decide if you want to look at it."

There are other ways this might be handled. If, for instance, another child's mother finds *Playboy* and says to her child:

Mother:	Where did you get this filthy magazine?
Child:	I found it.
Mother:	Where?
Child:	I can't remember.
Mother:	You are lying. Where did you get it?
Child:	I don't know.
Mother:	Go in your room and stay there until you tell me where you got it from.

What is the *basic message* regarding sex? It is that *Playboy* is a dirty magazine, the child is bad for having it, and anyone is bad for having it.

What was the *specific message* this mother got across to her child?

"You have done something very bad and I don't believe what you're saying. I will force it out of you because I am bigger and I have the power in this relationship."

Another approach by the mother could be: "I found a *Playboy* magazine under your bed. You are too young to be looking at this. I am taking it away. If it belongs to someone who should have it back, you can tell me and I will give it to the person."

What is the *basic message* regarding sex in this scenario? "*Playboy* is for older people." What was the *specific message* the parent got across to the child. "I don't want you to have this magazine at your age. I will give it back for you."

Another approach could be for the mother to say:

"I don't like these kinds of girlie magazines. When you are a grown-up you can decide if you want to look at them, but not when you're still a child living in my house. I am taking it away."

What is the *basic message* regarding sex? "I don't like girlie magazines in my house and especially for children to see." What was the *specific message* the mother got across to the child? "I don't like this type of magazine in my house and I am taking it away."

Now that you understand that there are a variety of messages that you may be conveying to your children, you can hopefully have clear, helpful conversations with your child. The next chapter will offer examples of actual conversations you can have with your child regarding sexual behaviors.

CHAPTER 11

Conversation Tips

Grace and Fred are middle-class parents who were devastated by Sam, their eleven-year-old next-door neighbor, engaging their five-year-old son, Michael, in sexual behaviors. Grace remembers the boys setting up a tent in the family room and playing "dead" inside the tent. What she didn't know at the time was that when one of the boys "died," the game was to touch the person they killed on the private parts over their clothes.

On another day when they were playing during this same time period, Sam encouraged Michael to touch his penis and his bottom with his hand when Sam pulled down his own pants. On a third occasion during the same several week period, Sam got Michael to give a quick kiss to his penis and asked Michael if he would like Sam to kiss his penis. Michael said "no." Sam didn't ask ever again.

Michael eventually revealed the touching incidents with Sam. Fred took Michael in his arms and said, "You did the right thing to tell us, we're proud of you." Michael's face brightened dramatically as if the weight of the world had lifted from his small shoulders.

When confronted, Sam immediately acknowledged the sexual behaviors with Michael, and together with his parents, came over to apologize. Sam said he should never have done that with Michael. He also told Michael that if ever again anyone tells him not to tell his parents something, that is the time when he should tell his parents. Michael accepted the apology and said he didn't tell his parents because he was afraid they would be mad at him.

While Grace and Fred were initially able to control their reactions, they soon panicked. With so much publicity about sexual abuse and the notion that victims become perpetrators, both parents started imagining the worst possible outcomes for Michael.

With no personal experience, both parents thought that sexualized behavior during childhood could cause severe damage to Michael in later life. In Fred's mind his son had lost his innocence and he feared that he would grow up to be a homosexual. "It's hard enough to grow up in this world, but if he is homosexual . . ."

Grace despaired that Michael would start touching other children. Since she found out about the incidents with Sam, Grace hadn't allowed Michael to play with other children unless she supervised him and the other child at her house. The parents' worries took over their ability to think clearly and they started telling Michael over and over again that he mustn't touch other children's "privates."

After a family visit to relatives Michael wet the bed. Grace asked him why he did that. He didn't know but related a dream he had. In the dream he had touched his cousin on his private parts. He asked his mother, looking fearful, whether she was mad at him. Without asking any more questions she said, "That would be a very bad thing to do. We've talked to you about this." He looked ashamed.

Incidents too numerous to describe began arising where Michael felt unsure of himself and would go to his parents to ask if he was doing the right thing. Most of the questions had to do with some kind of physical contact between himself and another person. A few were regarding private parts and others related to accidentally running into someone or getting squished in an elevator and touching someone. Virtually every other day he became highly concerned about physical contact he had with someone. He began to closely observe his friends and grown-ups and ask about physical contact between them. He always wanted to know when something was "bad."

Within a few months Michael came home visibly shaken saying he'd seen the penis of a classmate. Without asking anything further, his mother started to admonish him for looking at the child's penis. Seeing Michael made so distraught by his mother's response, Fred asked Michael to relate to him what had happened. After hearing the story of boys using a urinal and Michael seeing another boy's penis, his father told Michael there was nothing wrong with that and that he shouldn't worry. "That is normal." Michael looked relieved but soon became agitated several days later when he saw a man's penis when he was with his father in the bathroom at a movie theater.

As the parents related the history of interactions between Michael and Sam and the subsequent incidents related to touching and observations of genitals to their psychologist, she began to develop a hypothesis. Perhaps Michael's parents' fears about early sexual experiences between children had been transmitted in such a way as to make Michael feel like a bad child? Had he somehow come to blame himself for the contact with Sam? Did Michael think he was bad to have thoughts about private parts? Was his fear of being bad actually creating the thoughts about private parts to reinforce that he was bad? Had Michael developed a fearful, almost phobic reaction to physical contact with others, thoughts about private parts, and the observation of genitals, based on the parents' fears that he would develop "out-of-control deviant sexual impulses"? What messages were they giving Michael? What messages did they want to give Michael? What did they really believe about Michael's sexual development? What were the relevant facts and what were their fears?

As this was discussed during the consultation the parents got very worried that they had "ruined" their son. The psychologist tried to calm Fred and Grace. Children are very resilient and, yes, a course correction was in order. It was suggested that the parents decide exactly what they wanted to teach their son. Besides no physical contact with private parts, what values were they trying to teach? How did they want him to feel about sexuality? What feelings did they want him to have regarding physical contact with others? What did they consider sexual touch and what was child's play? Did they think some type of sexual exploration or contact between children was natural and healthy, and if so, how were they going to impart that to him?

Children can only take in a small amount of information at a time. Short, specific learning periods are the best. Repetition that is lighthearted is the key to success. Remember that rote learning regarding the acceptable norms of physical contact between children may bring no learning at all. When a child is anxious about a subject such as Michael was, he doesn't learn helpful information. He learns two things. Touching is bad and he is bad for doing it. He might also develop an urgent sense of "wanting to touch" to confirm that he is "bad." Read the following dialogues for tips on how to have these conversations with your child.

Mom: Any questions today about touching other people? (If you don't raise the subject, he may not. The idea is to keep up the learning and not only respond when he's anxious about some type of touch. When the parent raises the issue the child knows that the subject is always open for discussion.)

Michael: No. (Very few children will answer yes, don't worry, this is how children operate.)

Mom: Okay. I have an idea, let's talk about something you asked about before. Remember when you told Dad and me about a time at school when you saw Paul's penis. Remember that?

Michael: Yeah, you and Dad were really mad about that.

Mom: Oops. Dad and I weren't really mad, we were just worried. (When it comes to subjects about sex and sexualized physical contact, parents' fears often come across as anger to children.)

Michael: Why were you worried?

Mom: Let's remember what happened. (This is a good approach so you are sure you both remember the situation the same way. If he's operating on different facts, the conversation may mean something very different to him.) Tell me what you remember about that time.

Michael: I was at school in the cafeteria. Paul was sitting with his legs like this (knees bent with his feet up on the chair and his legs spreads apart) and his underwear was baggy and his "thing" was showing.

Mom: Yes, I remember that but I thought you said you asked him to spread his legs apart so you could see his penis. (It's best to use proper terminology.) Do I remember that wrong? (This is one of the critical junctures of the conversation. If you're sure Michael asked him to do it, say it in a questioning way, it allows Michael to take some responsibility and not be pushed in a corner to defend himself.)

Michael: Well, yes, I did want to see his penis but he started it.

Mom: How did he start it?

Michael: He was sitting like that and I could see inside his pants.

Mom: Oh, I understand a little better. I thought you asked him to open his legs like that so you could see his penis. (It's not essential that your version be correct. You're helping Michael learn what is important.) I didn't know he was already doing it. I think it would be different if you had asked him to open his legs. What do you think?

Michael:	Yeah, I wouldn't ask him to do that. He was already doing it and I thought it was funny.
Mom:	What do you think about Paul opening his legs so everyone could see his penis?
Michael:	It's nasty.
Mom:	Why is it nasty?
Michael:	'Cause think if a girl was around.
Mom:	Why would that make a difference?
Michael:	Girls shouldn't see boys' penises.
Mom:	Why not?
Michael:	It's a private part.
Mom:	I agree, but are penises only a private part between girls and boys?
Michael:	Hmm. I don't know.
Mom:	Tell me how you think we could decide?
Michael:	I don't know (sounding frustrated).
Mom:	Let's figure that out another time. For now I'm glad to understand the "penis sighting" (if possible, find some way to lighten up the conversation and make a little joking phrase that you can use again to make your point). Daddy and I didn't understand what happened. We thought you asked Paul to open up his legs so you could see his penis. I think that it's not all right to ask someone to do that. Now I understand that he was doing it and you pointed it out and thought it was funny. Maybe you helped him to remember to keep his legs together when he has on baggy underpants. Showing other people your private parts in a cafeteria is not okay. It would be different if everyone was changing their clothes and people saw each other's privates. Let's figure that out another time.
Michael:	Okay.

On another day Michael's father Fred tries to help Michael make sense of nudity.

Dad:	Let's try to figure out about seeing people's private parts.
Michael:	Yeah.
Dad:	Is your penis always your private part?

Michael:	Yes.
Dad:	What happens if someone sees some else's penis?
Michael:	It's gross.
Dad:	Always?
Michael:	Yeah, it's gross.
Dad:	Do you mean penises are gross? All boys and men have one.
Michael:	Penises are sort of gross and no one is supposed to see them. They're nasty.
Dad:	I don't understand what you mean.
Michael:	Me neither.
Dad:	Penises are part of a boy's body and a man's body, they aren't gross, they're useful. Let's think of a time when people might see someone else's penis.
Michael:	In the bathroom?
Dad:	Yes. You mean like when guys are using a urinal together.
Michael:	Yeah.
Dad:	How about other times?
Michael:	When they're changing to go swimming?
Dad:	Yes. How about other times?
Michael:	If they're changing clothes or taking a shower together.
Dad:	Yes. How about other times?
Michael:	I can't think of any others.
Dad:	Of the times you mentioned when guys might see each other's penis, when using the urinal, changing clothes, and taking a shower together, is there anything wrong about this?
Michael:	I don't know.
Dad:	What might make it wrong?
Michael:	I don't know.
Dad:	Let's think. If you were changing clothes and someone was peaking in a window at you and you didn't know it, would that be all right?
Michael:	No.

Dad:	I agree that is sneaky and that's not all right. Well then, when might it be all right?
Michael:	If my friends and I were going to go swimming and we were in my room changing, if I just looked over and saw Tommy's penis would that be okay?
Dad:	What do you think?
Michael:	I think it would be all right.
Dad:	I agree. You aren't sneaking and you aren't asking him to take off his clothes. He is just taking off his clothes to change for swimming. I don't see what could be wrong with it.
Michael:	Why were you and Mommy so mad when I saw Paul's penis in the cafeteria?
Dad:	We weren't mad but we were concerned because we thought you'd asked him to show you his penis. I don't think we should ask people to undress for us to look at them. If everyone is changing and you see each other naked, that is fine. No one is asking or forcing the other to take off their clothes in order to look at their naked body. Do you see a difference?
Michael:	Yeah, sort of.
Dad:	Let's try another example. Let's say your friend is changing his bathing suit on the beach. Someone is holding up a towel so he'll have privacy. Another boy comes along and rips down the towel. The boy tries to grab for the towel to cover up his naked body because he feels embarrassed. Is that all right?
Michael:	No, because he was trying to be private and not show his penis and someone is forcing him.
Dad:	Exactly, you got it. It isn't being naked and having your penis seen that is the problem. It has to do with where a person is, when it is, and whether the child is free to decide for himself if he is comfortable with being naked.
Michael:	I sort of get it.
Dad:	Any questions.
Michael:	Not really.
Dad:	Let's talk again.

The previous conversation may be hard to follow for a five-year-old child who is not struggling with the particular issues discussed. When a child is interested he or she will be able to follow the conversation. To assure that your child understands, listen carefully to what he or she says in response to your statements. Always try to use people and situations that are familiar to your child. It helps them understand.

One the day Michael comes to Mom looking ashamed and guilty:

Michael: I wanted to touch Grandma's bottom. Am I bad?

Mom: Tell me more about it.

Michael: I don't know anymore.

Mom: Where were you when you got this feeling?

Michael: Devon and I were joking about how fat it looks and then we were whispering about whether her bottom feels like marshmallows because she looks all puffed up (small giggle).

Mom: So what was your worry?

Michael: Am I bad because I wanted to touch her bottom?

Mom: What do you think?

Michael: I don't know.

Mom: Did you touch her bottom?

Michael: No, I wouldn't do that.

Mom: Why not?

Michael: That wouldn't be nice.

It is important for the parent to make sure he or she understands the correct details of what happened. After Grace understood what had actually occurred she was able to gather further information without making a quick judgment. Grace realized several things after listening carefully to what Michael was saying. Michael and a friend were teasing about grandmother. Since Grace had a brother she knows how boys giggle together and get in mischief. While the part of grandma's body he wanted to touch was the bottom, it had no sexual connotations. If she thought of the incident from the point of view (and height) of a high-spirited six-year-old boy and his cousin, the weightiness of the situation changed dramatically. She was concerned about sexual contact. He was squished in the elevator with a protruding bottom.

At this point Grace wants to tell him he shouldn't even be think-ing these thoughts. She wants to lecture him about making fun of people who are overweight, etc. She restrains herself knowing that the problem she and her husband are trying to undo regards Michael's belief that he is a bad person for wanting to touch someone. She is aware he is six years old and that she needs to focus on one problem at a time. Michael needs to know it is not all right to touch someone's bottom. The rest she can teach him by example and at other times as the situations arises. Right now she needs to bolster his ability to make decisions about physical contact with others.

Helping Children Talk to You about Sex

You're not the only one who has a hard time talking about sexual topics—your children also find it difficult! The following suggestions are for your kids. You may want to copy this page and give it to your child with an encouraging smile.

- Kids, even though it's hard to talk to your parents about sex-ual things, try! Here are some tips to help you.

- Some kids find it easiest to talk to the same-sex parent.

- If your parents come to you and want to talk, do it. You may want to run, but try to stay and listen. It probably took a lot of courage on your mom or dad's part to come to you! Don't make it any harder on them!

- You may be shy or feel like laughing when talking to your mom or dad about sexual things. Don't worry, they felt the same way when they were young.

- When you decide you want to ask a question about sex, don't ask it while your mom or dad is busy doing something else (like taking care of a younger child, vacuuming, trying to pay the bills, fixing the plumbing, etc.).

- If your mom or dad never seem to have time to sit down and talk to you, tell your parent/s that you would like to talk and ask when a good time would be.

- Remember, there are a lot of things to know about sex and sexuality. It's good to know how your body works and to understand all of the feelings in your body. It's also important to talk about your feelings about being sexual with someone else. When is it all right to do sexual stuff with other people? Your parents probably have ideas about that. Most parents like it if you would ask them your questions.

• If your parents says it's never okay to touch anyone in a sexual way, ask them when it will be all right. Ask them how they made the decision when they were young.

• ASK, ASK, ASK. If you want your parents' opinion about something, ask. You can't guess what they think. For instance, perhaps you wonder why many people say nasty things about homosexuals. Perhaps your parents have made comments you don't understand or agree with. ASK.

• If you're confused about something you heard, it's much better to check it out with your parents than stay confused. Other children usually don't know any more than you do, but they may make something up because they want you to think they know it all! Usually answers from grown-ups are more true.

• If you want to know how your parents handled sexual feelings and urges when they were your age, get up your courage and ask. Remember—they love you and want to help you.

• If it's information you want, ask specific questions. If you think your parent is getting stuck on an answer, suggest getting a book and reading it together.

• Ask your parents for some books about sex and sexuality that are good for kids your age.

• Sometimes children are worried about how their parents feel about them if they have been abused. Ask them, don't make up the answer yourself.

• Good communication about sex and sexuality takes practice. If your parents aren't so good at it, they can probably learn!

• If you can't talk to your parents about sex, ask them for another adult who they trust with whom you can talk. If you don't feel comfortable with their first choice, ask again. Getting an adult's ideas about sex and sexuality can be very helpful as you grow up.

CHAPTER 12

How to Reduce the Risk of Abuse to Your Children

Prevention programs have proven to be beneficial to children. Just ten or fifteen years ago there was little information available. Previously, few victims of sexual abuse knew how to identify or put a name to what was happening to them. Sexual abuse was hidden and children rarely spoke up. If they did there was no well-developed system to assist them. There were no treatment programs for sex offenders or victims. Although we have a long way to go, we have come a long way.

Most children are now aware that it's not acceptable for others to touch their private parts. They also know to tell someone. This will reduce the risk for many children from ongoing abuse. Sex offenders no longer operate in a society that is unaware of their presence. They have to be more devious and select their victims more carefully in order to avoid detection. Prevention information has provided an understanding to children and to adults who are now more aware of sexual abuse and know how to respond to children when they tell.

Understanding Sexual Abuse

Yet there are different kinds of sex offenders. There are those who abduct children they don't know to abuse. This is a very small group of sex offenders, probably less than 5 percent, but they get the most attention. Although this is an extremely small group of offenders most prevention programs teach children how to avoid this type of offender. Children are told to shout "no" and run and tell an adult. However, the majority of sex offenders don't operate like this. They're manipulative and befriend children and, in most cases, they know their families. Sex offenders may also be opportunistic. They may simply take advantage of a situation where there is a child they think they can take advantage of without being caught, without previously befriending them.

As our knowledge of sexual offending has increased and prevention programs become more sophisticated, children are no longer told that offenders wear raincoats and hide behind trees. Material has been incorporated that makes children aware that it may be someone they know, even a family member. Most sexual offending is done by a family member or someone well-known to the child. Sexual abuse by strangers is uncommon.

Certain programs now include information on adolescents being potential offenders. Approximately 40 percent of sexual offending to children is done by adolescents. Few programs include information on children forcing other children into sexual behavior. While children do molest other children, the majority of problematic sexual behavior between children is sexually-reactive behavior or children engaging in extensive but mutual sexual behavior. (See chapter 6.)

Children and parents need to understand the way sex offenders operate. Without an understanding of how child molesters offend, children and adults often believe they will be able to identify a sex offender by knowing they're out there. This isn't the case. Sex offenders are generally indistinguishable from the public at large. They don't look different than anyone else. Yet, there are many ways that child molesters act that can help parents detect them.

After the discovery of a pedophile who molested many boys in Canada, the eleven-year-olds were asked, "Why didn't you tell?" The boys said no one ever told them that "a sex offender would make friends with us and be really nice, thoughtful, and kind."

How Most Sex Offenders Operate

Although there are many types of sex offenders there are two types that commit most offenses against children. There is (1) the sex offender who takes time to "groom" the victim, and (2) the opportunistic sex offender who takes advantage of a situation in which there is a vulnerable child. They are both highly manipulative.

The offender who "grooms" develops a relationship with the child. It's only after a period of engaging the child in a pleasant or need-satisfying emotional relationship that the offender begins to engage in some form of physical contact with the child. Only after the offender involves the child in a fair amount of emotionally and physically pleasant touch does the offender begin the sexual behavior. These offenders may be family members or people outside of the family. While most sexual offenders are men, up to 10–15 percent may be teenage girls or women.

The opportunistic offender takes advantage of situations. There may be little or no "grooming" (establishing the relationship and setting up the child for being vicitimized). The offender simply takes advantage of a situation in which there is a child they believe is vulnerable. Adults and adolescents engage in opportunistic or situational offending. For example, David, age ten, went to swim practice. He got there early and was waiting for his team to arrive. The janitor asked him if he would like to see the machinery and filters used to keep the pool clean. He had seen the janitor many times and because he was bored he went with him to look. While in a back room, the janitor asked him to pose for some photographs for a commercial he was making of special kids. David agreed. The offender made the picture-taking fun. He encouraged David to make lots of faces and clown around.

Next the offender, the janitor, asked David to pull down his swimsuit for a photograph of his bottom. "This will be a really funny picture," said the offender. The offender saw David's reluctance but encouraged him by saying he wouldn't take a picture of his face. David got uncomfortable but went along with it to get out of there. David got scared when the offender wanted to take a picture of his genitals from the front.

As the offender was trying to back down because he realized he'd made the child uncomfortable, David said, "I'm sure my team is here, I have to go." The offender realized that he had scared the child and hence the child might tell. The offender then said "This is our secret. Remember, I have the photographs and you agreed to them." David ran out of the swim complex.

Since abuse by an opportunistic sex offender took place quickly with little or no buildup, it left David off balance. Children often just want to forget that it ever happened. Some children do this successfully, others remember but don't tell, and others tell. The following section offers ways to increase the likelihood of a child getting out of an offending situation and telling after it occurs.

Developing a Relationship with the Parents

If the sex offender isn't a family member, he or she may develop a relationship with the parents first, or at least meet them in order to gain their trust. Some of these offenders already hold a position of trust by being a minister, priest, choir master, music teacher, tennis or soccer coach, and so on. The offender may sound very open, inviting the parents to come to his or her home or go on outings together. By the contact with the parent, the child molester may be trying to determine the parents' work schedule and likelihood to drop by his or her house unannounced.

The child molester may also want to get a sense of the relationship between the parent and child. Does the parent have the time to meet the child's needs for comfort and love? Does the child seem to need more companionship? Is the parent so overwhelmed with stressors that he or she or both parents may welcome someone to spend time with the child? Does a single mother feel her child needs a male in his or her life? Does a single father think his or her child needs a female in his or her life?

In front of the parents the offender may reassure them about his or her strictness with the child regarding maintaining rules and boundaries. This reassures the parent and also provides a cover if the child complains about something. Thinking that the offender is strict, the parent might think the child just doesn't like the offender's strictness. The offender may want to assess the closeness of the relationship between the parents and child to determine the parent's likelihood to listen to and believe the child, rather than the adult, if the child should say something about the sexual interaction.

The offender may want to assess the sexual mores and attitudes of the parents and get a sense of the boundaries in the home. The looser the boundaries around sex, sexuality, and privacy in the home, the more susceptible the child is to the offender engaging in intrusive behaviors with the child and the child not realizing what is happening.

For instance, if the child doesn't have privacy in the bathroom at home, the child will not be surprised if the sex offender goes into the bathroom with the child or allows the child in the bathroom with the offender. If sexual material is left around the child's home or there is a great deal of overt sexual expression in the home, the child will not be surprised if that happens with the child molester. If the parents aren't very responsive to the child's requests that they stop doing something like drinking or swearing, or tickling them, the child will not be surprised or think to tell their parents (and expect them to respond) if the offender does these things.

Confusing the Child

It can be a long time before a child realizes the offender is doing something wrong. The younger the child, the longer it takes for him or her to become aware that something is wrong. Very young children may never figure it out. This is dependent on several things. If the offender only plays games that are fun for the child such as "magic wand" (offender to child, "See how many ways you can make the wand stand up") a child under five or six may never realize that it's wrong.

These games are only sexual to the offender. If the offender never causes the child any physical pain, monitors the child's reactions to the behavior, and never goes beyond the child's comfort level, the child may not realize there's something wrong. Some children don't realize something is wrong until they begin to talk to their friends and discover that not all daddies or mommies, aunts, uncles, grandparents, or neighbors play these games with children.

For the child who does figure out that something is wrong, he or she has likely been in an emotional relationship with the offender for a period of time and will not want to hurt his or her feelings. Those who have some unmet emotional needs may not want to lose the positive emotional relationship to the offender. It's also hard for children to question adults' behavior and authority. We teach children to do what the grown-ups tell them. Many children who are abused by a family friend or relative are told when they leave the house with the adult, "Do what he (or she) tells you." Sometimes a parent might even say something like, "I don't want to get a bad report about you."

Because the sexual behavior is only a part of the relationship, some children decide to "put up with it" in order not to lose the emotional relationship. The sexual behavior is generally not understood by young children as sexual or abuse. They don't understand the meaning of this behavior to the adult. Children usually want it to be over with, particularly if there's any genital contact involved. Most offenders don't physically hurt children, which sometimes facilitates the children's choice not to risk losing the emotional relationship.

A factor that further complicates the disclosure of abuse is that offenders encourage the children to believe that they want the relationship, including the sexual contact. "You like this, don't you. You have fun when we are together." "When you come to me, we have fun." "I can tell you like the presents and fun we have together." Offenders make children feel responsible for all aspects of the relationship. Children then feel it's their fault and that they'll be in trouble if they tell.

Many sex offenders diminish the child's love and dependence on their parents. They encourage the child to rely on them. They try to make the child feel that their parents (or the other parent in incest situations) don't care about them as much as they do.

Children often don't trust that their parents or another adult will believe them if they tell. This can be because it would be their word over an adult's. Offenders reinforce this belief by such statements as "Your mother won't believe you if you tell her. She will believe me, not you. Who will she think is lying? Your mother trusts me."

Many sex offenders make the child feel responsible for keeping them safe. "If you tell anyone about our secret you will ruin my life." "I could go to jail." "You will ruin our family." "It will be your fault if there is no money to take care of the family after I am in jail." This makes some children feel they must take care of the offender and that the offender's safety is more important than taking care of themselves.

Physical Responses

Children who have been sexually abused may have felt some physical or sexual (genital) pleasure from the abuse. Approximately 20 percent of children twelve and younger feel sexual stimulation (as an adult might feel) during their childhood. Around 32 percent of children who have been sexually abused report feeling sexual stimulation (as an adult might feel).

When children feel pleasant feelings in their genitals or sexual stimulation (as an adult might feel) it can be more difficult for them to assign blame to the offender. They may believe the only reason the sexual behavior is happening a second time is because they liked what the offender did to them. Offenders reinforce the idea that it's the child who wants the sexual contact and, in many cases, makes the child believe it's their fault.

This frequently produces feelings of guilt, shame, and confusion in the child. Children can rarely see through or understand how they are manipulated by the sex offender. One of the most durable beliefs of the sexually abused child is that it was his or her fault.

Children are caught in a terrible bind. Disclosure of sexual abuse is extremely difficult for them if it's by a manipulative sex offender or by the opportunistic sex offender who is also manipulative. If there is physical force or physical pain involved (regardless of whether or not there was ever any sexual stimulation) it's far easier for children to disclose (if they're safe from the offender) and much easier for them to determine who is at fault. In any case, ongoing sexual abuse by a family member or people who are well-known to the family is difficult for children to disclose because of the way sex offenders develop relationships with their victims.

Innoculating Children Against Manipulative Sex Offenders

Children who are the most vulnerable to long-term abuse by sex offenders are those who don't know about natural and healthy touch and who don't understand their rights regarding what people can say and do to them. Children who don't have any practice understanding how they think and feel, knowing how to express themselves and to whom to express themselves, may be the targets of sex offenders and others who will take advantage of them.

Although probably no children are risk free, children who have secure relationships with one or more adults and live in stable environments have the least susceptibility to ongoing abuse by sex offenders. In the secure relationship the child's needs for caring and comfort are met and the child is listened to as well as being allowed to question adults.

Children who live in these homes know that if they make a mistake, they'll still be loved and will have an opportunity to explain their side of the situation. It is essential that you teach your children their rights. This entails respecting the children's rights and modeling respect between all members of the family. Children who grow up knowing their rights and the responsibilities of others to them, have the best chance of evading sex offenders.

Raising Healthy Children Who Know Their Rights

In some families, children cannot question adult authority. "Do as you are told." "Do it because I said so." "I am the adult and what I say goes." Children who are allowed to ask questions and express themselves when they're uncomfortable will more naturally question situations that seem incorrect. Children who are not given free reign to think through their relationships to others and openly discuss things that concern them, lack important skills to evade sex offenders. Children cannot make the rules, but they can ask for them to be explained. Endless explanations and reexplanations by parents to children are not warranted. But at least one explanation at the level the child can understand is warranted.

It is important to respect your children's emotional, physical and sexual space. Privacy for bathroom use, changing clothes, and whatever other private times the child wants should be provided. Their bodies should be respected. If they don't like kissing all of their relatives, don't make them. It's a perfect opportunity to teach them: "I know Aunt Tilly and don't think there's any reason not to kiss her, but it's your body. You can make decisions for yourself about how you want to use it. Just stick out your hand right away and shake her hand."

If your child still lets Aunt Tilly kiss him or her, intervene. Say, "Aunt Tilly, Jeff (or Suzie) feels a little uncomfortable about kissing you. I want him to know he can make those choices. Do you mind if you two shake hands or do high fives?" Medical needs can be handled differently. "I will be with you if any doctor needs to touch your private parts. We'll talk about it with the doctor if that needs to happen. No one has a right to touch you anywhere unless you agree to it."

Set Clear Examples

The best way to teach your children is by clear examples. From an early age allow your children to have certain toys that are theirs alone. They have control over these special toys. If they don't want others to play with them, that's their choice. Just like their toothbrush, there are some things that are theirs alone. Teach them that the toys and their toothbrush are just like their body. They make the decisions.

This should also extend to being tickled. If a child doesn't like to be tickled, the parents can reinforce that it's his or her right to make that decision. "Even though I like to tickle you, I'm glad you tell me what you like and don't like. I won't do it if you don't want me to." Don't go into the bathroom when someone else is using it. Knock; if your child says come in, go in. If your child wants privacy, give it to them. These strategies teach children their rights. It also teaches them the rights of others. If you need privacy they must give it to you. (There are exceptions when young children need supervision.)

As your children are growing up, you're educating them about a million things. Again, a part of this process should be teaching the proper names for all of their body parts. Include the names for private parts. When children have names for the parts of their bodies, they're more likely to speak about them. Specific names for the vagina, penis, bottom, and nipples are good for children to learn while toddlers. Elementary school children can learn labia, testicles, clitoris, scrotum, shaft and head of the penis, and so on.

Children who are used to using the words for their genitals and hearing their parents use them are more likely to feel comfortable to speak with their parents, if some problem arises. If your children have never spoken to you about their genitals, they're far less likely to than if they feel comfortable talking about these parts of their body. Some parents like to use nonstandard words. While this is certainly up to you, it's not a good idea to use negative names like "nasty" related to sex or sexual parts.

If children's needs for affection, caring, comfort, and safety are met within the family they will be far less vulnerable to manipulative sex offenders. Children who have a positive sense of their ability to make judgments, think about problems, and use the adults around them to ask for advice are far less likely to be targeted by sex offenders. Sex offenders often target children who have few friends, seem troubled, and whose parents are overburdened and have little time for them.

A family that communicates comfortably about easy as well as difficult subjects is fundamental to reducing the risk to the child from the manipulative sex offender. Children who are afraid of their parents' punishments will be less likely to tell their parents if they are fooled by a sex offender into sexual behavior. When children feel confident that even if they did something wrong they can go to their parents and be given a chance to explain, they are more likely to take the chance and tell their parents.

If you give punishments that don't follow logically from your child's misbehaviors, he or she will not be able to anticipate what you'll do in a specific circumstance. But when your child knows that you'll listen and be fair if he or she goes to you with a problem, your child is far more likely to tell you. Yet, children feel very trapped by sex offenders. Even with a healthy and happy home life a child can fear telling his or her parents about a nonfamilial sex offender or an offender in the extended family. If the offender is a parent, the home life is not without problems or ongoing incest could not occur.

Parents should watch for signs of change in their children's behavior. Since all children react differently, there aren't universal signs to watch for—but *any* signs of change in the child's moods, behavior, or relationship to parents or others should be noted. When a child says he or she isn't happy at the day care, with the baby-sitter, at school, etc., take it seriously. Sit down and listen to whatever your child has to say, then investigate. Children need to know they will be taken seriously.

Specific Inoculations Against Sexual Offenders

The following suggestions are to assist you in reducing the risk of abuse to your children. Although they may seem scary, they're impor-tant points. Children can be given many tips, but sex offenders are devious. You are the primary protection for your children. Besides raising emotionally healthy children, you can do the following:

- Be aware of new people (adult or adolescent) who come into your life or the life of your child who want to develop a rela-tionship specifically with your child. Most manipulative sex offenders want to spend more time with your child than you would expect. If there's a significant age difference between the new person and your child, be cautious.

- Be aware of people in your children's lives who take a large interest in them. While no parent wants to be overly protec-tive, it's often the person the parents know well who sexually abuses their children. Coaches, teachers, Boy and Girl Scout leaders, church leaders, baby-sitters, nannies, boyfriends, people you allow to spend a lot of time at your house, hus-bands, wives, aunts, uncles, grandparents, etc., all have a great deal of access to your children. Unfortunately you must be aware of any person who may take advantage of your children. The largest percentage of offenders to children are stepfathers.

- Be aware that sex offenders may target single parents with children of the age and gender they prefer to molest.

Offenders believe that single parents will have less time to spend with their children therefore making the children more susceptible to the "affection," "caring," and time the offender has available to give.

- Be aware of people who want to do a lot of things for you when you'll not be at home and your child will be with that person. Be aware of people who offer to baby-sit, or clean or fix something in your home while your children are there alone.

- When your child is with someone about whom you have any concern, let the adult know you *may* drop by where they are, even if you're not going to do it that very day. But, do drop by on occasion, if you have any reason for concern. Children should have the telephone number where you can be reached.

- Watch and listen to your children's reactions to being with people with whom you leave them. If you see any hesitation, or overenthusiasm to be with the other person, or a secretiveness about what goes on, this may signal something is wrong. Check in with your child about this. Remember "the something wrong" could be a lot of things, including spending a lot of money on the child, doing drugs, drinking, having pornography around, or permissiveness about rules. While these are harmful in themselves, they can also be a lead-up to sexual abuse. Offenders often give "forbidden" things to children that the children like and want but can't have at home because of the cost or because you will not allow it. When the children realize that this person is a sex offender, they are afraid to tell because of having accepted the "forbidden" things. They fear that you will be mad.

- Tell your children how offenders entrap children. Remember to tell your child at the level he or she can understand, making sure you don't scare them but only alert them. This will help them recognize it, if it should happen. In talking to your children about the possibility of someone mistreating them, make sure they're aware that when something occurs that is different from what they expect, either at home or when they're away from home, they should question it. Encourage your child to talk over things with you that they think are "kinda different or kinda strange or 'iffy.'"

- Speak casually to your child if you're concerned about something: "Anything going on with Dick (Jane) that you think is different from what you might expect?" "Anything different from what goes on at home?" "I am always available if you are worried about anything or just want to talk." "Remember, I won't be mad if you tell me something you think may be a problem. We will just talk and find a way to solve your worry."

- Let your child know they can always tell someone "we don't do that at home and my mom (dad) would be mad if I do that here. I don't want to." When your child is leaving home with someone, instead of saying, "Do as Dick (Jane) says," say, "You know how we act here and what our rules are, do the same with Dick (Jane).

- Listen carefully to your child about his or her outside activities. Don't just do it on the run. Child molesters are some of the best listeners, this is one of the ways they make children feel cared about. Children will frequently drop small hints to their parents if they are worried. A hint is far more likely than a full description or direct statement of any concerns or abuse. Keep your ears open for the hints.

- Make sure your children know all of the people they can tell if they are concerned about anything that happens outside their home. There are people at school, church, day care, and everywhere children are to whom they can talk when they are concerned. Assure that your child knows to keep telling until something happens. Children can also tell school counselors or therapists or others when there are things going on at home that concern them.

- Be aware of your child's behavior and moods. The best way to detect that your child is having a problem or worried about something is by a change in behavior or mood that persists beyond the one or two day "moody" phase of children.

Boundaries

People need their own emotional, physical, and sexual "space" and must respect others' space. One of your tasks is to teach your children about their own rights to *personal space* and *physical privacy* as well as the rights of others. This assists your child in knowing when a sex offender is crossing the expected boundaries.

Parents generally teach their children the rules regarding privacy. Yet, in some families, people don't have a right to physical privacy or the rules may change depending on who is in charge or whose privacy is being protected. Adults usually have the right to privacy in their bedroom and in the bathroom. While children old enough to care for themselves should also have privacy, this isn't always the case. Children are often confused about privacy because of the lack of clarity in their homes. Children who are clear about their rights to privacy know when a sex offender is violating those rights.

Privacy is one issue related to physical boundaries. Another is an individual's right to his or her personal space. Personal space is an invisible area around an individual that doesn't have a definite measurement but the person knows when it's being invaded. Personal space is less an issue among children than among children and adults. Children roughhouse, sit squeezed together in cars, or piled on top of each other while watching TV. As children develop, the amount of personal space they require expands. Infants hug the adult's body, toddlers are carried, preschool children hold the parent's hand, elementary school children may walk side by side, and the teenager walks on the opposite side of the street from their family!

You Are the Personal Space Teacher

Your children learn about personal space from you and the adults who interact with them. Some parents aren't aware that they may not be teaching their children about their right to personal space. They may hug the child longer than the child wants to be hugged and chide the child for trying to squirm away. Parents may shower with the child long after the child requires help and after the child feels comfortable with the nudity.

You need to pay attention to your child's needs and desires for personal space. This will teach your child that this is what he or she can expect. When you listen to your child's discomfort he or she will expect this from others. Some parents persist in assisting children with their personal hygiene long after the children can take care of themselves. This is the same type of intrusion into the child's personal space in which an offender engages. If parents do this to their children, the children don't know their rights and will not know when an offender is "grooming" them to prepare them for sexual behaviors.

The outcome of not teaching personal space requirements can be children who also don't understand the space requirements of others.

Children who run right up to people and get in their face to talk to them, grab their arm, sit on their lap, ask for a hug from unknown people or people with whom they don't have a relationship, are violating others' physical space. They don't know when theirs is violated or when they're violating someone else's.

Sex offenders may target these children. Offenders sometimes test the children's boundaries. For instance, he or she may touch their hair, then later their shoulder and arms, then their back, etc. Each time the offender can test to see if the child will move away in discomfort. Children who don't move away are more likely to remain the targets of sex offenders. Sex offenders don't want to be caught—so they stay away from children who are more likely to tell or be strict with their boundaries.

Emotional boundaries are violated when a person cannot have private thoughts and when others' feelings are projected onto them. When there are role reversals in the home, the children's emotional boundaries are disregarded. In some families with poor boundaries children are placed in the role of protector of a parent. This can mean that they're told the details of the parents' problems, and become the friend or confidante of the parent. Sexual boundary violations include children being told the sexual intimacies of the parent, being put in the role of the surrogate boyfriend or girlfriend, observing intimate sexual behaviors by the parents, and being encouraged to act in sexually seductive ways or being sexually touched. If children think this is acceptable behavior, they're not alerted to the sex offender who may also do any or all of the above. If children expect this type of behavior or think it's how adults are, they'll not be alerted to something being wrong when a sex offender does this.

Internet Dangers

On the Internet there are vast numbers of people making contact with each other. There are advertisements for pornography, strip shows, and sex paraphernalia that are available when email is delivered. There appears to be no way at this time to stop these from entering the home. Children have access to them as easily as adults.

Unfortunately, the Internet is another avenue for child molesters to find vulnerable children. You need to monitor your children's time on the Internet. The chat rooms can be dangerous places for children. They can be exposed to sexual conversations that are way beyond their capacity to understand. There have been reported cases of child molesters making contact with children on the Internet and meeting them off-line. Children need to be aware of the dangers on the Internet. As with everything, if your child feels comfortable talking with you, he or she will be less likely to be searching out other adults with whom to share experiences. As with television, videos, magazines, and other forms of communication, you need to be aware of your child's interests and guide them in healthy directions. The wealth of information on the Internet is staggering. You can "surf the Net" with your child and point them in positive directions.

Children—Be Aware

There are many things that will be valuable for you to tell your child. The following list includes some of them. These are the content—you will need to translate them for the age and level of understanding of your children.

- If you're ever worried that something is wrong about the sexual things going on in your home or anywhere else you are, ask us—your parents. If you are still concerned, your school counselor, pastor, or teacher may be good people to ask.

- If you feel uncomfortable with what someone is saying to you about sex, tell them so and/or excuse yourself, and *leave*.

- If you don't like something one of us or someone else does that has to do with sex and sexuality, tell him or her. You probably should start off gently and always respectfully. For instance, perhaps you see someone do a lot of kissing and touching. You can say, "Mom (Dad, George, Sarah), I don't like it (it makes me feel uncomfortable) when you do all the touching in front of me. Could you do that in private?"

- If an adult or adolescent lets you get away with things that you know are wrong and that we wouldn't be okay with, watch out. Why would they do this? Maybe they want something from you. There is a saying: "If something is too good to be true; it's usually too good to be true." BEWARE.

- "If something is too good to be true, it's usually too good to be true" is also a good motto when surfing the Net or talking in chat rooms. Child molesters contact kids on the Net. You cannot tell a child molester from anyone else on the Net; don't think you can, even the professionals can't. Don't agree to meet anyone you met on the Net. Don't give them your name or address.

- If anyone is telling you about a sexual relationship they have with another person and you feel uncomfortable, say, "I'm uncomfortable when you talk to me about that stuff. Please don't."

- If anyone is using sexual language or talking about sexual things that make you uncomfortable, you can say something like, "I'm uncomfortable when you talk that way. Please don't." You can also just make an excuse and leave.

- If you feel uncomfortable with the way someone is touching you anywhere on your body, move away. If they continue, ask them to stop and/or get up and move away. If you're not sure if it's all right for the person to do that, trust your instincts and judgment. If you don't like it, you have a right to not have it happen. [Children do have to have some medical procedures, but you'd be present for that.]

- It isn't just touching the private parts that you have a right to ask to be stopped, it's any type of touch that is unpleasant to you or makes you feel "weird" or uncomfortable.

- If you feel unloved and need some more hugs and kisses, ask for them or give them to us yourself. This will help us remember to give them to you.

- Compare how people treat you and how they treat other children. Be aware of what you like and don't like. Don't feel that anyone has a right to treat you unkindly. Speak up. If you can't get them to change, ask someone to help you.

- If someone is trying to get you to join in a conversation about sex or use sexual language with which you're uncomfortable, you can say, "No thanks, I've got to go." You can also just make an excuse and leave.

- If someone is trying to get you to do something sexual you don't want to do or don't think you should do, you can say, "I need to call my mother. She told me to call her about this time." You can also just make an excuse and leave.

- If you don't like pictures or videos that someone wants you to watch, you can say, "I'd rather watch television." You can also just make an excuse and leave.

When You Think Your Child May Have Been Abused

If you suspect anything, be calm, don't overreact. Children need support. If they feel there is any possibility of you being mad at them or hurting the other person or making them go talk to the other person, they may immediately make up an excuse to retract.

If you feel you need clarification, make sure your questions are open-ended. Don't ask specific questions that require "yes" and "no" answers or ask about specific people unless the child has named a specific person. If, while you're asking nondirect or nonspecific questions your child uses a name, you can then use it. (Be sure to clarify to whom the child is referring if he or she does give a name. There are lots of "coaches." The child may have several people he or she calls "dad," there may be three Steven's in his or her life, or the person may have the same name as a friend of yours but be a different person.)

The questions you probably need answered are the "wh" questions. Who, what, when, and where. "Why" isn't a good question because the child will not have an answer for that, nor would we. The safest method to use to gather information in order not to get incorrect information is to keep your mind open and try not to lead the child to say something in particular or someone in particular (you have already guessed) is the problem or the culprit.

For instance, if your child comes home and says his penis hurts, don't panic. In a calm and caring manner:

You: Your penis hurts?

This statement is to clarify that you heard the child's statement correctly and to show the child that you're not panicking, accusing anyone, or getting upset in any way. This will help your child continue. Wait for child to respond.

You: When did it start to hurt?

Wait for child to respond.

You: Do you know what might have happened to start it to hurt?

Wait for child to respond.

Child: John touched my pee-pee.

You: John touched your pee-pee.

This statement is said matter-of-factly to clarify that you heard it correctly. Raise your voice slightly at the end of the sentence indicating that you want a confirmation of what he said.

You: Tell me some more about John touching your pee-pee.

Your son tells you that it happened in the bathroom after a soccer game. John was touching his penis while he was trying to go to the bathroom. John said he was just trying to make sure his penis was all right. Your son told John to stop it because he didn't like him rubbing it up and down. John told him not to tell anyone or that John wouldn't be able to be the coach anymore and their team would lose the season.

Talking to Your Child

Any further information you might ask is only to determine if there is a reasonable or logical explanation for your child's statements other than inappropriate sexual contact. As soon as you believe you have enough to be suspicious of abuse, call the police if the alleged offender is not a family member. If the alleged offender is a family member you can call the police or the Child Abuse Hotline. The operator can give you the telephone number. Remember, parents are not investigators. Parents or anyone who *suspects* abuse can call the Child Abuse Hotline. Investigation should be left to the professionals.

Remaining calm and matter-of-fact, tell your child that adults should not touch children's pee-pees (use the child's own words) and that you will call someone to help figure out what to do about it. Let your child know that you are sorry that it happened, proud that he told you, and that you love him. *Give him a hug and a warm proud smile* and ask if there is anything else he wants to talk about right then. Let him know that if he doesn't want to talk more now, that anytime he wants to talk about John or what happened or anything else you'll be always ready to talk to him.

Try very hard not to convey the message indirectly that the child should have or could have stopped the touching from happening. Be aware not to question why a child didn't tell earlier, if the molest happened some time ago. While this is hard for parents not to do, it's beneficial to the child who most likely struggled to tell when he or she did. The answer to the question will most likely become known after the investigation and when the child is more comfortable. Often when the child discusses how the abuse took place it will be evident why the child told when he or she did and not earlier.

It's extremely difficult for parents when they discover their child has been victimized. Anger, fear, dismay, sadness, hurt, a desire for revenge, and guilt are but some of the reactions they may experience. Try to keep your strong reactions out of the sight and hearing of your child. Parents are often more affected by single or a few incidents of nonpenetrative and nonphysically assaultive sexual abuse than young children. If the child sees or hears the strong reactions, he or she may feel the need to take care of the parent's anguish. Children can misinterpret a parent's strong reaction as being a result of something they did wrong or evidence that they're damaged. Be careful that your children are not privy to any of your adult discussions, either overhearing something when you're on the phone or when the child is with you.

What Can You Do?

Research supports that one of the most important variables that determines the outcome for children who have been sexually victimized is the response of the adults when the abuse is disclosed. Children need to feel loved, cared about, comforted, understood, listened to, and supported when they disclose abuse. When the child's parents are able to provide this support, effects will be lessened, particularly if the child lives in a consistent, caring, predictable environment where he or she feels safe.

Most helpful is for you to listen carefully to any and all concerns of your child and not guess how he or she feels. Children have many different responses to being a victim of sexual abuse. Your response should be in direct response to the needs of your child. Don't assume your child's response is the same as yours—this would be rare. Remember, your child is unique. The situation the offender set up and the abuse that occurred is unique, your child's experience of the abuse is unique. There are no standard responses of children to sexual abuse. Listen to your child.

Remember that sexual abuse is an event. It has been found that it's not necessarily the event but the child's, and parents', *reaction* to the event that predispose him or her to develop symptoms. You can be a powerful force in your child's perception of the event. If you see your child as damaged and portray this to your child, this may affect him or her. Since the effects of events are different for different children, have your child assessed. Do not predetermine what the effects are.

You need to be observant and listen carefully to your children at all times. This doesn't change or begin because your child has experienced sexual abuse. While it's helpful to be observant and listen to your child it's not helpful to worry. This can lead to your behaving differently. Parents who think victims of sexual abuse become perpetrators sometimes act differently toward their child. This can include not touching, hugging, cuddling, wrestling, or kissing the child; watching all of the child's actions expecting negative behaviors; and looking for disturbed sexual behaviors. This can be very detrimental to a child's sense of self and can increase the child's feelings of "being bad" or "damaged goods" after abuse.

In this regard a study of teachers in elementary schools is important to note. Teachers were given children with equal capabilities but some were told the children had high capabilities and others were told their students had low capabilities. The test scores of the children mirrored the belief systems of the teachers.

You can also have a powerful effect on your children's growth and development. If you think your child is damaged, he or she may also believe this. Again, the point is to assess your child accurately and not have preconceived ideas about the outcomes. Listen to your child and help him or her with whatever is needed.

Getting Help

Most parents and children need guidance from someone familiar with the reporting of abuse and the steps that are followed after a child's disclosure of sexual abuse. You can call the Child Abuse Hotline and ask for advice. This can be done anonymously, if you want to get information before you make the actual report. After the police and/or Child Protective Services have responded you can ask them for advice. They can help you as well as provide mental health referrals. Parents need assistance to manage their feelings and know how to support their child. This is true in extrafamilial abuse, as well as when the sex offender is a family member.

Sometimes, when the abuse was: a one time (or very few times) occurrence; the child disclosed the abuse; it was nonpenetrative and nonassaultive; and *not* by a family member; and you see no changes in your child's behavior or feelings; and you feel confident to help your child, you may want to seek advice from a professional and use this advice to help your child. Parents who can be supportive of their child and who are able to talk openly with their child about the abuse may be the majority of the help the child needs. Ongoing mental health intervention with the child is not always needed. In general though it's best to have a mental health professional who is experienced in working with sexually abused children evaluate your child. In this way you will feel confident that a professional assessment has been done and the professional can determine if therapy is required. Your child will know that that person is available if any worries or concerns come up about the sexual abuse that you can't help with, or which the child would rather discuss with the therapist.

If you and your spouse or partner disagree with one another about whether the abuse actually occurred, are in conflict because the (alleged) perpetrator is one of your parents or a relative, or your child from another relationship, or you have a conflictual relationship prior to the abuse, you should get the help of a mental health professional who is experienced in the treatment of sexual abuse. Since parents are focal to the best outcome for the child after abuse, parental discord can be highly detrimental to the successful resolution of the abuse for the child. Unfortunately, some parents cannot give up their own needs and arguments for the best interest of their children. If this is a problem for you or your partner or spouse you'll need help quickly.

If you or your partner or spouse feel that the abuse should *never* be discussed with your child, you will also need the help of a mental health professional. The therapist will help you speak to your child or, in the event that you cannot, help the child understand why. Whereas ongoing discussion of the abuse may not be necessary, it's unwise for a child never to discuss it with their parents and to feel that it's a taboo subject. This decreases the child's comfort in dealing with what happened to him or her, decreases the probability that he or she will tell if it happens again, and leaves the child questioning what is so bad that it cannot be discussed. This can lead the child to think he or she is bad, or speculate about other reasons. Open dialogue when it's helpful to the child is most healing. Children should not be left with unanswered questions.

If you are so upset by the abuse that you're afraid you might cry or breakdown if you speak to your child, you should get the assistance of a therapist for you and for your child. With help you will be able to talk to your child. In the meantime, your child will talk to the therapist. Both you and your partner or spouse should be open to speaking to your child about the abuse at the times when it's in the best interest of your child.

Therapy

Children may need help to sort out what happened to them. Some children will not recognize that what happened was abuse. If a child enjoyed the attention, the child may miss the offender and feel upset that he or she told. If the child felt sexual arousal, he or she may have enjoyed this and want more or feel guilty for experiencing this. If the offender was a parent or relative the child may feel it's his or her fault that the family is fighting or disrupted.

There are many things that can cause confusion for a child. This can be worked on in individual therapy. For some children group therapy with other same-age children who have suffered similar abuse is best. This can help the child know that other children get abused and that they don't look any different after this happens. Knowing they are not the only one and talking to other children with similar experiences can be beneficial.

When a child who has been sexually abused requires therapeutic intervention, the parents will also benefit from working with a therapist. Virtually all parents will need help if their child has been abused. There are a million feelings that arise. Was it my fault? Why didn't he tell me? I should have known something was wrong. I brought the offender into the house because I wanted attention. It's my fault she was abused. You need someone to help you answer your questions and to help you help your child. If the perpetrator was a spouse, partner, or your own child, you will need a great deal of help. It's hard to get any perspective when the abuse is done by someone you care about to someone you care about.

In some cases the parents and child can have the same therapist. In other cases a different therapist will be better. Whether multiple therapists are required will depend on many factors and should be decided by the child's therapist. Working with the parents of the child who has been abused is one of the most essential needs for assisting the child who has been sexually abused. The parents' response to the child's disclosure of abuse and their ongoing interactions to assist the child to heal are critical factors in the successful outcome for sexually abused children. The therapeutic needs of the child's parent/s will be different depending on whether the abuse was by a spouse or partner, or by a relative, or by someone outside the family. In all cases, therapeutic work with the parents is essential. The experienced professional will guide the parents and child to a healthy resolution.

When there have been multiple forms of abuse or disruption in the child and family's life, these will also require therapeutic intervention. In some cases there may be a need for a medical examination for gathering evidence or to rest the parents' and/or child's mind that the child's body is fine.

Some Facts about Child Abuse

What is the incidence of child abuse in the United States?

In 1997 there were 1,054,000 *confirmed* cases of child abuse in the United States. This represents about one-third of all of the cases reported to authorities as *suspected* child abuse. In other words, about one-third of all suspected child abuse cases were confirmed. This represents about fifteen out of every 10,000 children in the United States. This means that approximately 1.5 percent of children in the United States are *confirmed* victims of child abuse each year.

It is quite certain that this is an underestimate of the actual occurrence of child abuse as this is only what comes to the attention of authorities.

What is the incidence of the different types of child abuse?

In 1997 there were 84,320 cases of confirmed sexual abuse; this was 8 percent of all confirmed cases of child abuse. This is approximately .1 percent of all children in the United States.

Physical abuse constituted 22 percent of the confirmed cases; neglect 54 percent; emotional abuse 4 percent; all other forms of abuse 12 percent.

Are there many children molested in day care centers?

There has been a fear amongst parents that there is a substantial amount of sexual abuse in day care centers in the United States. David Finkelhor, one of the finest researchers on child abuse in the United States, studied the reported instances of sexual abuse in day care centers between January 1983 and December 1985. The incidence was approximately 500–550 cases in a three-year period, which included 2500 victims. This is approximately 5.5 victims per 10,000 children in out-of-home care. This was less than the number of children sexually abused in their homes, which was estimated at 8.9 victims per 10,000 children under six years of age (Finkelhor 1986).

Is there a lot of sexual abuse in the out-of-home care of children?

Data is available for the occurrence of sexual abuse in day care centers, foster care, and residential facilities that care for children. The incidence for confirmed sexual abuse in all three types of out-of-home care for children was approximately 2 percent of all confirmed cases in eighteen U.S. states. This 2 percent rate was constant for the eleven years prior to and including 1995 (Lung and Daro 1995).

What is the most frequent age for confirmed cases of child abuse?

Children who are the most vulnerable, or at least about whom we know the most, are children seven to twelve years of age. To get information on child abuse go to www.childabuse.org

Computer Scoring for the Child Sexual Behavior Checklist (CSBCL)

The CSBCL can now be computer scored for easy analysis of a child's sexual behaviors. Treatment planning is greatly simplified by receiving a printout of the type, frequency, and severity of the child's sexual behaviors, and a ranking of any problematic characteristics of the child's sexual behavior, as described by his/her parents/caregivers. The responses of multiple parents/caregivers can be analyzed separately or compared so that similarities and differences in their perception of the child's sexual behavior can be noted. Decisions on the level of severity and the child's primary sexual problems are provided.

The following will also be included in the computer generated report:

- Are there certain sexual behaviors which are important to evaluate very carefully?

- Which of the child's current sexual behaviors may make him/her more vulnerable to a child molestor?

- Which sexual behaviors were previously observed but are not currently being observed?

- Are there notable differences between respondents' observations of the same child's sexual behavior?

The CSBCL costs $4.00 for a copyrighted original, which can be duplicated with the author's permission. To order send request to the address below. Carefully follow the directions regarding how to complete the CSBCL. Keep the original and send a COPY of the CSBCL, $6.00, and a self-addressed stamped 9x12 envelope. A ten to fifteen page report will be sent to you.

> CSBCL Computer Scoring
> Toni Cavanagh Johnson, Ph.D.
> 1101 Fremont Avenue, Suite 101
> South Pasadena, CA 91030

Research Participants

One study described in this book was completed by 394 college students from eight different two- and four-year state colleges throughout the United States. An anonymous questionnaire was given to the students in class. The same information regarding the research, giving a thorough description of the study, and that it was voluntary, was given to each class prior to administration of the study.

Each student was asked for his or her permission to use the study results. Those who agreed signed a release form. The questionnaire asked about their sexual behaviors when they were twelve years old and younger. Forty-four percent of the students who completed the questionnaire were male and 56 percent female. An average of 80 percent of students who were provided the questionnaire completed it. Their average age was twenty-five years old.

Sixty-one percent were Caucasian, 18 percent Hispanic, 4 percent African-American, 16 percent Asian, and 1 percent were unclassified. Seventy-three percent were single, 24 percent married, 3 percent divorced, and 1 percent separated. Ninety-nine percent were heterosexual, .5 percent homosexual, and .5 percent bisexual. Forty-three percent were Catholic, 40 percent Protestant, 2 percent Jewish, 3 percent Buddhist, 1 percent Muslim, 1 percent Fundamentalist, and 10 percent had no religion. The mean income was middle to lower middle class.

A second survey of 352 mental health professionals and child welfare workers has also been used to describe children's sexual behaviors. This data was gathered at the beginning of training sessions given by the author on the topic of children with sexual behavior problems throughout the United States. As participants entered the training they were given a one-page questionnaire and asked to fill it out, if they were willing. The questionnaire was anonymous. A box was available for them to hand it in during the first break. The sample was 81 percent female and 19 percent male. Their average age was thirty-nine. No other demographic data were gathered.

References

Achenbach, T. M. 1983. *Manual for the Child Behavior Checklist and Revised Child Behavior Profile*. Burlington, VT: University of Vermont.

Alexander, M. 1999. Sexual offender treatment efficacy. *Sexual Abuse: A Journal of Research and Treatment*. 11(2): 101–116.

Ascione, F., and P. Arkow, Eds. 1999. *Child Abuse, Domestic Violence and Animal Abuse—Linking the Circles of Compassion Prevention and Intervention*, Purdue: University Press.

Cooper, M., and Haynes. 1996. Characteristics of abused and non-abused adolescent sexual offenders. *Sexual Abuse: A Journal of Research and Treatment* 82:105–119.

Finkelhor, D. 1981. Sex between siblings: sex play, incest and aggression. In *Children and Sex*, edited by L. Constantine and F. Martinson. Boston: Little, Brown & Company.

Finkelhor, D. 1986. *A Sourcebook on Child Sexual Abuse*. Beverly Hills: Sage.

Friedrich, W. 1997. *Child Sexual Behavior Inventory Professional Manual*. Odessa, FL: Psychological Assessment Resources, Inc.

———. 1998. Behavioral manifestations of child sexual abuse. *Child Abuse and Neglect* 22(6):523–531.

Friedrich, W., and J. Fisher, et al. 1998. Normative sexual behavior in children: A contemporary sample. *Pediatrics* 101(4).

Friedrich, W., and W. Luecke. 1988. Young school-age sexually aggressive children. *Professional Psychology Research and Practice* 19(2):155–164.

Gil, E. and T. C. Johnson. 1993. *Sexualized Children: Assessment and Treatment of Sexualized Children and Children Who Molest.* Rockville, MD: Launch Press.

Hanson, R. K., and Slater. 1991. Characteristics of sex offenders who were sexually abused as children. In *Sex Offenders and Their Victims*, edited by R. Langevin. Oakville, Ontario: Juniper Press.

Haugaard, J. J., and C. Tilly. 1988. Characteristics predicting children's responses to sexual encounters with other children. *Child Abuse and Neglect* 13:209–218.

Johnson, T. C. 1988. Child perpetrators—children who molest other children: preliminary findings. *Child Abuse and Neglect* 12:219–229.

———. 1989. Female child perpetrators: Children who molest other children. *Child Abuse and Neglect* 13(4):571–585.

———. 1989. Female child perpetrators: Children who molest other children. *Child Abuse and Neglect* 134:571–585.

———. 1990. Important tools for adoptive parents of children with touching problems. *Adoption and the Sexually Abused Child.* J. McNamara, and B. McNamara, Human Services Development Institute University of Southern Maine: 75–88.

———. 1991. Understanding the sexual behaviors of young children. *SIECUS Report* August/September.

———. 1993. Assessment of sexual behavior problems in preschool and latency-aged children. A Yates, Ed. *Child and Adolescent Psychiatric Clinics of North America.* Philadelphia: Saunders.

———. 1997. *Sexual, Physical, and Emotional Abuse in Out-Of-Home Care, Prevention Skills for At-Risk Children.* New York: Haworth Maltreatment and Trauma Press.

———. 1998 *Treatment Exercises for Abused Children and Children with Sexual Behavior Problems.* South Pasadena, Calif.: Self-published.

——— 1998. Child sexual behavior checklist-revised. *Treatment Exercises for Abused Children and Children with Sexual Behavior Problems.* South Pasadena, CA: Author.

——— 1998. *Sexuality Curriculum For Children and Young Adolescents, and Their Parents.* South Pasadena, CA: Author.

———. 1998. *Treatment Exercises for Abused Children and Children with Sexual Behavior Problems.* South Pasadena, CA: Author.

———. 1998. *Understanding Children's Sexual Behaviors—What's Natural and Healthy and What's Not?* South Pasadena, Calif.: Self-published.

Johnson, T. C., and C. Berry. 1989. Children who molest other children: a treatment program. *Journal of Interpersonal Violence* 4(2): 185–203.

Johnson, T. C., and C. Friend. 1995. Assessing young children's sexual behaviors in the context of child sexual abuse evaluations. *True and False Allegations of Child Sexual Abuse Assessment and Case Management*. T. Ney. New York: Brunner/Mazel.

Kaufman, J., and E. Zigler. 1987. Do abused children become abusive parents? *American Journal of Orthopsychiatry* 57(2):186–192.

Kendall-Tackett, K. A., L. Williams, et al. 1993. Impact of sexual abuse on children: A review and synthesis of recent empirical studies. *Psychological Bulletin* 113(1):164–180.

Lung, C., and D. Daro. 1995. *Current Trends in Child Abuse and Fatalities: The Results of the 1995 Annual Fifty State Survey*. Chicago, Illinois: National Committee to Prevent Child Abuse.

Milloy, C. 1998. Specialized treatment for juvenile sex offenders: A closer look. *Journal of Interpersonal Violence* 13(5):653–656.

Morgan, S. R. 1984. Counseling with teachers on the sexual acting-out of disturbed children. *Psychology in the Schools* 21 (April):234–243.

Perry, B. D. (in press). Incubated in terror: Neurodevelopmental factors in the cycle of violence. In *Children, youth. and violence: Searching for solutions*, edited by J. D. Osofsky. New York: Guilford Press.

———. 1993. Neurodevelopment and the neurophysiology of trauma I: Conceptual considerations for clinical work with maltreated children. *APSAC* 6(l):14–18.

———. 1994. Neurobiological sequelae of childhood trauma: Post-traumatic stress disorders in children. In *Catecholamine Function in Post-Traumatic Stress Disorder: Emerging Concepts*, edited by M. Murberg. Washington, DC: American Psychiatric Press: 233–255.

Piaget, J. 1971. *The Construction of Reality By The Child*. New York: Ballantine.

Rind, B., P. Tromovitch, R. Bauserman. 1988. A meta-analytic examination of assumed properties of child sexual abuse. *Psychological Bulletin* 124(1):22–53.

Sirles, E., J. Smith, and H. Kusama. 1989. Psychiatric status of intrafamilial child sexual abuse victims. *Journal of the American Academy of Child & Adolescent Psychiatry* 28:225–229.

Wang, C. T., and D. Daro. 1998. *Current Trends in Child Abuse Reporting, and Fatalities, The Results of the 1997 Annual Fifty States Survey*, Chicago, Illinois: National Committee To Prevent Child Abuse.

Weeks, R., and C. Widom. 1998. Self-reports of early childhood victimization among incarcerated adult male felons. *Journal of Interpersonal Violence* 13:346–361.

Widom, C., and M. Ames. 1994. Criminal consequences of childhood sexual victimization. *Child Abuse and Neglect* 18(4):303–318.

More New Harbinger Titles
for Parents and Families

KID COOPERATION
How to Stop Yelling, Nagging, and Pleading and Get Kids to Cooperate

There really is a way to talk so that kids will listen and be reinforced to be helping, responsive members of the family. This is an empowering work, filled with practical skills.

Item COOP $13.95

WHY CHILDREN MISBEHAVE
And What to Do About It

This text offers practical strategies for dealing with common behavior problems in a concise, easy-to-use format. Beautifully illustrated by over 100 photographs.

Item BEHV $14.95

WHEN ANGER HURTS YOUR KIDS
A Parent's Guide

Learn how to combat the mistaken beliefs that fuel anger and how to practice the art of problem-solving communication—skills that will let you feel more effective as a parent and let your kids grow up free of anger's damaging effects.

Item KNOW $12.95

THE POWER OF TWO
Secrets to a Strong & Loving Marriage

Details the skills that happy couples use to make decisions together, resolve conflicts, recover after upsets, and convert difficulties into opportunities for growth.

Item PWR $15.95

COUPLE SKILLS
Making Your Relationship Work

A book that can change your relationship—by changing how you communicate, how you think about your partner, how you behave, and how you cope with problems and conflicts.

Item SKIL $14.95

Call **toll-free 1-800-748-6273** to order. Have your Visa or Mastercard number ready. Or send a check for the titles you want to New Harbinger Publications, 5674 Shattuck Avenue, Oakland, CA 94609. Include $3.80 for the first book and 75¢ for each additional book to cover shipping and handling. (California residents please include appropriate sales tax.) Allow four to six weeks for delivery.

Prices subject to change without notice.

Some Other New Harbinger Self-Help Titles

Claiming Your Creative Self: True Stories from the Everyday Lives of Women, $15.95
Six Keys to Creating the Life You Desire, $19.95
Taking Control of TMJ, $13.95
What You Need to Know About Alzheimer's, $15.95
Winning Against Relapse: A Workbook of Action Plans for Recurring Health and Emotional Problems, $14.95
Facing 30: Women Talk About Constructing a Real Life and Other Scary Rites of Passage, $12.95
The Worry Control Workbook, $15.95
Wanting What You Have: A Self-Discovery Workbook, $18.95
When Perfect Isn't Good Enough: Strategies for Coping with Perfectionism, $13.95
The Endometriosis Survival Guide, $13.95
Earning Your Own Respect: A Handbook of Personal Responsibility, $12.95
High on Stress: A Woman's Guide to Optimizing the Stress in Her Life, $13.95
Infidelity: A Survival Guide, $13.95
Stop Walking on Eggshells, $14.95
Consumer's Guide to Psychiatric Drugs, $16.95
The Fibromyalgia Advocate: Getting the Support You Need to Cope with Fibromyalgia and Myofascial Pain, $18.95
Healing Fear: New Approaches to Overcoming Anxiety, $16.95
Working Anger: Preventing and Resolving Conflict on the Job, $12.95
Sex Smart: How Your Childhood Shaped Your Sexual Life and What to Do About It, $14.95
You Can Free Yourself From Alcohol & Drugs, $13.95
Amongst Ourselves: A Self-Help Guide to Living with Dissociative Identity Disorder, $14.95
Healthy Living with Diabetes, $13.95
Dr. Carl Robinson's Basic Baby Care, $10.95
Better Boundries: Owning and Treasuring Your Life, $13.95
Goodbye Good Girl, $12.95
Being, Belonging, Doing, $10.95
Thoughts & Feelings, Second Edition, $18.95
Depression: How It Happens, How It's Healed, $14.95
Trust After Trauma, $15.95
The Chemotherapy & Radiation Survival Guide, Second Edition, $14.95
Surviving Childhood Cancer, $12.95
The Headache & Neck Pain Workbook, $14.95
Perimenopause, $16.95
The Self-Forgiveness Handbook, $12.95
A Woman's Guide to Overcoming Sexual Fear and Pain, $14.95
Don't Take It Personally, $12.95
Becoming a Wise Parent For Your Grown Child, $12.95
Clear Your Past, Change Your Future, $13.95
Preparing for Surgery, $17.95
The Power of Two, $15.95
It's Not OK Anymore, $13.95
The Daily Relaxer, $12.95
The Body Image Workbook, $17.95
Living with ADD, $17.95
When Anger Hurts Your Kids, $12.95
The Chronic Pain Control Workbook, Second Edition, $17.95
Fibromyalgia & Chronic Myofascial Pain Syndrome, $19.95
Kid Cooperation: How to Stop Yelling, Nagging & Pleading and Get Kids to Cooperate, $13.95
The Stop Smoking Workbook: Your Guide to Healthy Quitting, $17.95
Conquering Carpal Tunnel Syndrome and Other Repetitive Strain Injuries, $17.95
An End to Panic: Breakthrough Techniques for Overcoming Panic Disorder, Second Edition, $18.95
Letting Go of Anger: The 10 Most Common Anger Styles and What to Do About Them, $12.95
Messages: The Communication Skills Workbook, Second Edition, $15.95
Coping With Chronic Fatigue Syndrome: Nine Things You Can Do, $13.95
The Anxiety & Phobia Workbook, Second Edition, $18.95
The Relaxation & Stress Reduction Workbook, Fourth Edition, $17.95
Living Without Depression & Manic Depression: A Workbook for Maintaining Mood Stability, $18.95
Coping With Schizophrenia: A Guide For Families, $15.95
Visualization for Change, Second Edition, $15.95
Angry All the Time: An Emergency Guide to Anger Control, $12.95
Couple Skills: Making Your Relationship Work, $14.95
Self-Esteem, Second Edition, $13.95
I Can't Get Over It, A Handbook for Trauma Survivors, Second Edition, $16.95
Dying of Embarrassment: Help for Social Anxiety and Social Phobia, $13.95
The Depression Workbook: Living With Depression and Manic Depression, $17.95
Men & Grief: A Guide for Men Surviving the Death of a Loved One, $14.95
When Once Is Not Enough: Help for Obsessive Compulsives, $14.95
Beyond Grief: A Guide for Recovering from the Death of a Loved One, $14.95
Hypnosis for Change: A Manual of Proven Techniques, Third Edition, $15.95
When Anger Hurts, $13.95

Call **toll free, 1-800-748-6273,** to order. Have your Visa or Mastercard number ready. Or send a check for the titles you want to New Harbinger Publications, Inc., 5674 Shattuck Ave., Oakland, CA 94609. Include $3.80 for the first book and 75¢ for each additional book, to cover shipping and handling. (California residents please include appropriate sales tax.) Allow two to five weeks for delivery.

Prices subject to change without notice.